Health-Related Quality of Life in Cardiovascular Patients

Kalina Kawecka-Jaszcz • Marek Klocek •
Beata Tobiasz-Adamczyk • Christopher J. Bulpitt
Editors

Health-Related Quality of Life in Cardiovascular Patients

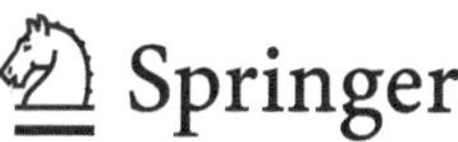

Kalina Kawecka-Jaszcz
Professor of Cardiology and Internal Medicine
I Department of Cardiology and Hypertension, Jagiellonian University Medical College, Kraków, Poland
e-mail: mckaweck@cyf-kr.edu.pl

Marek Klocek
Associate Professor of Internal Medicine
I Department of Cardiology and Hypertension, Jagiellonian University Medical College, Kraków, Poland

Beata Tobiasz-Adamczyk
Professor of Sociology
Chair of Epidemiology and Preventive Medicine, Jagiellonian University Medical College, Kraków, Poland

Christopher J. Bulpitt
Professor of Geriatric and Cardiovascular Medicine Experimental Medicine (Care of the Elderly), Division of Medicine, Imperial College London, Hammersmith Campus, London, UK
e-mail: c.bulpitt@imperial.ac.uk

Contributors
Bogumiła Bacior, **Leszek Bryniarski**, **Danuta Czarnecka**, **Magdalena Loster**, and **Katarzyna Styczkiewicz**
I Department of Cardiology and Hypertension, Jagiellonian University Medical College, Kraków, Poland

ISBN 978-88-470-5585-8 ISBN 978-88-470-2769-5 (eBook)

DOI 10.1007/978-88-470-2769-5

Springer Milan Dordrecht Heidelberg London New York

Softcover reprint of the hardcover 1st edition 2013

9 8 7 6 5 4 3 2 1 2012 2013 2014 2015

Cover design: Ikona S.r.l., Milan, Italy

Typesetting: Ikona S.r.l., Milan, Italy

Springer-Verlag Italia S.r.l., Via Decembrio 28, I-20137 Milan
Springer is a part of Springer Science+Business Media (www.springer.com)

Preface

This book provides a unique overview of quality of life (QoL) in cardiovascular medicine. It provides much information on QoL: in hypertension; in coronary artery disease and its treatment (with drugs and interventions); in heart failure; if there are disturbances in cardiac rhythm; if implantable cardiac devices are employed; in post-stroke patients. Thus, the book is useful for the practising physician, cardiac surgeon or stroke physician. Moreover, it is an invaluable resource for anyone considering research in these areas. In addition, the Appendix provides appreciable detail and full citations on generic and disease-specific QoL questionnaires.

We hope and expect that the book will help researchers to move forward in the scientific areas detailed above. There isout of necessary, an element of repetition, but we hope this is not excessive and helps to reinforce many important points.

The first chapter by Beata Tobiasz-Adamczyk sets the theoretical framework for QoL. She emphasizes that we limit the discussion of QoL to health-related Quality-of-Life (HRQoL), and that measures of QoL must reflect the views of patients rather than their carers. She predicts that HRQoL measures will be applied universally despite conceptual difficulties and theoretical uncertainties.

The second chapter, by Marek Klocek and Kalina Kawecka-Jaszcz, considers HRQoL in subjects with hypertension. They emphasize that QoL measures, although considered to be "soft" endpoints compared with biochemical or physical measures, must be scientifically determined, valid, repeatable, and provide quantitative data. The problem with reduced HRQoL in hypertension is that it may arise from: the disease; telling patients that they have hypertension (thereby engendering anxiety and adoption of a sick role); poor control of blood pressure despite treatment. The authors state that women are more likely to report impaired HRQoL than men, and discuss the HRQoL on different anti-hypertensive treatments.

The third chapter is by the same authors and considers coronary artery disease

(CAD). Very interestingly, in this condition (and probably other conditions) a poor measure of HRQoL predicts poor survival for reasons that have yet to be determined. Allowance for the severity of coronary heart disease, other co-morbidities, as well as psychological and demographic factors do not destroy this relationship. Factors improving HRQoL in CAD include a positive affect, rehabilitation, surgery for CAD, percutaneous intervention, and drug treatment. HRQoL in this condition is reduced by coronary pain, lack of social support, depression, and cognitive dysfunction (the latter being more common than expected in CAD). In young survivors with CAD, HRQoL is equivalent to the reduced QoL of the general population that is 20 years older.

Leszek Bryniarski and Marek Klocek, in the fourth chapter, discuss HRQoL in patients after percutaneous coronary intervention (PCI). They provide more detail on the effects of PCI and coronary artery bypass grafting (CABG) on HRQoL. PCI has been associated with better HRQoL than medical treatment over a 6–24-month period, but not after 36 months. This appears to be especially true in those aged > 80 years. There is evidence that HRQoL is improved with CABG rather than PCI, especially in men. “Off-pump” CABG improves HRQoL immediately after the procedure compared with conventional CABG, but long-term HRQoL appears to be identical in both procedures. The authors also discuss the use of bare-metal and drug-eluting stents as well as their use in acute coronary syndrome in the very elderly.

The fifth chapter is on HRQoL in heart failure (HF) and is written by Marek Klocek and Danuta Czarnecka. HRQoL is particularly poor in patients with HF. This is especially true if the individual: is young; is female; has a large burden of symptoms and severe restrictions on physical activity; has concomitant diseases: is under considerable stress. Interestingly, HRQoL in HF is not closely associated with ejection fraction. Beta-blockers do not improve HRQoL in HF, but sartans and ivabradine may do so, as may increased nursing support, intravenous administration of iron, and exercise.

The chapter on HRQoL with disturbances in cardiac rhythm is written by Bogumiła Bacior and Katarzyna Styczkiewicz. HRQoL in atrial fibrillation (AF) is dependent upon whether or not the condition is symptomatic and whether it is permanent rather than paroxysmal (the latter probably being associated with a less good HRQoL). There appears to be no evidence that electrical cardioversion improves HRQoL although radiofrequency ablation with subsequent pacing may do so, as may surgical treatment. In supraventricular tachycardia, ablation appears to be superior to pharmacotherapy for improving HRQoL. In vasovagal syncope, HRQoL is reduced but no drug therapy has yet to be shown to improve this situation.

Bogumiła Bacior and Magdalena Loster co-author the seventh chapter: HRQoL with implantable cardiac devices. A pacemaker improves HRQoL, and dual pacing may prove to be better than ventricular pacing. Pacemakers with a rate-response function reduce symptoms, and cardiac resynchronization therapy reduces mortality in HF and improves HRQoL (especially in those with severe HF symptoms). Implantable cardioverter-defibrillators reduce HRQoL during the first 6 months, often due to anxiety and especially if the device discharges. After this period, HRQoL does not appear to be high and, on average, is similar to that seen for amiodarone.

The last chapter, on HRQoL after stroke, is written by Marek Klocek. In this condition, HRQoL is dependent upon the degree of disability, psychological state (especially depression), cognitive functioning, communication difficulties and, most importantly, the level of independence. The QoL of carers is also reduced. When considering HRQoL after stroke, attention must be paid to fatigue and to pain (especially in paralyzed limbs), and to the effects of treatment (such as use of anticoagulants). Marek Klocek also provides a very useful table of HRQoL in various conditions. He concludes with an extensive and very useful Appendix on available questionnaires.

Christopher J. Bulpitt

Contents

The Genesis of Health: Evolution of the Concept of Health-Related Quality of Life

1

Beata Tobiasz-Adamczyk

1.1 Definition

Quality of life (QoL) was first introduced as a concept in medicine in the 1970s. In the 35 years that followed, it saw unparalleled growth, confirmed by numerous studies and scientific publications devoted to measuring QoL in different groups of patients subjected to specific medical interventions.

As applied to medicine, QoL arose from the social sciences. It was in this context that the term "health-related quality of life" (HRQoL) was developed to signify the QoL of an individual which resulted from his/her health status, experience of disease, and process of natural aging. The scope of this term points to various meanings in a medical perspective, and results in the need to reference different theoretical concepts and definitions which may be applied to specific medical specialties [1–5].

There has been a surge of interest in measuring HRQoL in patients diagnosed with various illnesses. Along with the expansion of medicine beyond purely traditional approaches, the results of treatment based only on biological criteria have become inadequate. Nowadays, clinical studies focusing on the effects of chronic disease more often go beyond biological measurements of health. Instead, clinical studies have a multidimensional approach in which special attention is paid to the emotional experiences, wellbeing, and potential for everyday functioning of patients [6]. In other words, attention is now also focused on the indicators of health that reflect the patient's ability to function in different areas of life [7–13].

Therefore, measuring QoL has gained special significance in reference to the long-term medical care of chronically ill individuals. It is also considered relevant if a return to health is only temporary and incomplete. As a result of the development or

B. Tobiasz-Adamczyk (✉)
Chair of Epidemiology and Preventive Medicine
Jagiellonian University Medical College, Kraków, Poland
e-mail: mytobias@cyf-kr.edu.pl

K. Kawecka-Jaszcz et al. (eds.), *Health-Related Quality of Life in Cardiovascular Patients*,
DOI: 10.1007/978-88-470-2769-5_1 © Springer-Verlag Italia 2013

progression of illness, symptoms may be exacerbated to an irreversible point where the patient might be a candidate only for palliative care [14].

According to Bowling [15], QoL serves as the endpoint of any measurement concerning the quality of medical services. It gives a subjective measure of health status from the perspective of the patient, and indicates the degree of his/her satisfaction with treatment or the results of treatment.

Presently, several researchers refer to QoL according to the definition developed by the World Health Organization Quality of Life (WHOQOL) Group. According to this definition, QoL is "the individual's perception of their position in life in the context of their culture and value systems in which they live and in relation to their personal goals, expectations, standards and concerns" [16]. In this context, QoL denotes a complex measurement of the health status of an individual. This measurement is inclusive of: physical health; emotional state; independence in life; level of dependence on one's environment; relationship with one's surroundings; and individual beliefs and convictions [16].

The definition of QoL has led to many problems in terms of conceptualizing and making the term operational. Researchers have observed significant differences in how this definition is applied in the determinants of self-rated QoL. Conceptualizing QoL may be done through a general evaluation of life satisfaction as well as by measuring more specific and detailed dimensions of this concept [17, 18].

Arnold et al. [19] applied a hierarchical model to conceptualize QoL that was developed on the basis of studies conducted by Spilker [20]. This model applies three conceptual levels to understanding QoL: from the most general (level I) to a level identifying indicators which may be used to measure different the dimensions of QoL (level III). According to this model, measuring general QoL is related to general life satisfaction and general wellbeing. Measuring general life satisfaction is tantamount to the measurement sought after by the WHO definition. The second level identifies different dimensions of QoL, which are most often inclusive of psychological, social, and physical functioning. At this level, certain authors also examined other dimensions of QoL, such as professional activity, economic status, individual productivity, degree of cohesion with one's surroundings, and the presence of chronic disease. These dimensions can be analyzed collectively or separately. Level III defines specific markers (i.e., indicators, aspects) which can be used to measure and identify each specific dimension. The model developed by Spilker assumes that the most detailed indicators of QoL (level III) significantly influence general QoL (level I). It would then be possible to determine the relationship between functional status and general QoL. In measuring functional status, the consequences of illness may be significant. This dimension may determine the measure of other dimensions or QoL in general.

In a critical analysis of the consequences of applying this model, Arnold et al. [19] noticed that general QoL is not always determined by changes in health status. This is because, in the course of their lifetime, individuals are exposed to several changes in their surroundings or to important life occurrences which affect them directly. As a result, individuals have to repeatedly adapt to different situations, which may stabilize the measure of general life satisfaction so that it appears to be fixed even in cases of altered health status.

If we accept that QoL should be defined as the ability to live a "normal" life, then the social determinants of this "normalcy" are accepted as active participation in all areas of social life, such as work, leisure time, family, and community activities. Subjective determinants include the degree of satisfaction with which individuals fulfill their physical, psychological, and social needs as well as their participation in social structures.

Self-rated QoL is dependent upon objective changes to health status, a stable personality, and individual predisposition. It is also dependent upon behavioral, cognitive, and emotional processes which support adaptation to change in health status, modification of goals, and developing accommodation strategies for everyday actions and behaviors. "Response shift" is of significant value in long-term measurements. This concept implies a change in the meaning which individuals ascribe to their QoL resulting from a modification of their internal standards and hierarchy of values.

Measuring QoL as the endpoint of treatment or of a particular time-defined intervention may lead to a change in response shift. This change results from a modification of self-defined constructs used to evaluate the endpoint (i.e., QoL). The first construct includes internal standards used by the individual in self-evaluation. The second construct represents the significance ascribed by the individual to different dimensions of the concept under evaluation or the varied importance of different dimensions of QoL (i.e., changes in the hierarchy of values of individuals). The final construct deals with redefining or changing the conceptualization of the concept itself (i.e., self-rated QoL).

According to Siegrist and Junge [21], studies examining QoL in chronic diseases are valuable sources of medical information because they supplement data from laboratory and diagnostic testing. By equating QoL with self-rated health status, Siegrist and Junge posited that QoL studies in medicine serve three functions. Firstly, they present the patient's viewpoint, which may be completely different from that represented by clinical studies and basic scientific research. The patient observes his/her illness from the perspective of his/her own psychosocial life situation and self-rated physical condition. Appropriate physician–patient communication as well as mutual cooperation in the healing process requires the physician to know how the patient rates his/her life situation relative to his/her health status. Secondly, subjective measurements by patients are an additional source of information which may prove valuable if making a therapeutic decision (especially if more than one treatment option may be used). Both may yield an identical result in a "biological" sense, but their impact on QoL may be different. Lastly, they may be indicative of how the physician fails to meet the needs of his/her patients. This is reflective of ensuring appropriate healthcare outside the hospital setting.

1.2 Reasoning Behind Introducing QoL to Medicine

Special interest in QoL first appeared in medicine in the 1970s and served to describe the health and non-health consequences of chronic disease. It also served to measure the clinical and non-clinical effects of physician interventions as well as general healthcare in areas as oncology, internal medicine (including cardiovascular diseases (CVDs)), geriatrics, rheumatology, and psychiatry. Interest in QoL was related directly to new approaches in measuring the effects of treatment not only through assessing longevity (e.g., after a particular treatment), but also by measuring the "quality" of the life which was extended as a result of successful therapy. This implied that longevity should be improved in a biological sense, and that such treatment options should be used that could ensure (i.e., after the illness, treatment, or in the course of therapy) a standard of living that was similar or identical to that of healthy individuals [5, 9].

At first, HRQoL was conceptualized as being based on a model of pathology and dependence. Thus, it focused on measuring reduced physical and psychological agility as well as dysfunctional fulfillment of one's social roles and functions. As a result, it was indicative largely of the negative consequences of restricted functioning.

Currently, HRQoL has been refocused to more "positive" measurements. Such measurements reflect the patient's ability to function in different life situations (even in the event of an untreatable chronic disease or disability). Measuring patients' HRQoL is dependent upon the acceptance of specific criteria. Firstly, chronic diseases often require long-term, continuous and, at times, dynamic accommodation to changes in one's ability to function in different areas of life. Secondly, chronic diseases also require the patient's family, immediate surroundings and society to assimilate to living with a chronically ill individual. Lastly, the consequences of illness require changes in behavior and the fulfillment of social roles. This includes role modification or, at times, the necessity to resign from a particular function.

In an analysis of patient adaptation to chronic disease, attention must be drawn to the role of time. This relationship is reflective of the time needed by the patient to reorganize his/her everyday activities as well as various changes. Specifically, this includes changes in: the disease over time and variations in social consequences; how the particular disease is perceived over time; how the relationship between the disease and social consequences is perceived over time.

It seems that some clinicians may have difficulty in accepting a measurement of HRQoL carried out by the patient. This measurement is often an expression of the patient's adaptation to his/her disease and a new hierarchy of values. It may also even be an entirely modified personal definition of HRQoL, a definition which would not have changed were it not for the disease. This internal mechanism of adaptation to disease (i.e., response shift) explains the often encountered paradox of high values of HRQoL in patients facing difficult clinical situations ("disability paradox").

1.3 Scales Used to Measure QoL

The increasing importance of QoL studies in clinical medicine is paired with the need to develop tools which adequately reflect the different dimensions of HRQoL. The requirements of such tools often differ from those of widely used functional scales, which tend to focus on patient-reported functional difficulties in areas of everyday physical, emotional, and social activity [22–25].

It is difficult to conceptualize HRQoL because of its multidimensional nature and the many aspects involved in its measurement. Applying the concept of QoL to measure the effects of medical interventions is dependent upon the definition used (i.e., the current health status and social determinants with which it is connected). Without such consensus, it is difficult to appropriately define what HRQoL is or how it should be measured [13, 26] (Table 1.1).

Table 1.1 Domains of Quality of Life

Pain and discomfort	energy and fatigue, sexual activity, sleep and rest and sensory functioning
Positive feelings	thinking, learning, memory, and concentration; self-esteem; bodily image and appearance; and negative feelings
Mobility	activities of daily living; dependence upon medicinal substances and medical aids; dependence upon non-medical substances; communication capacity; and work capacity
Social relations	practical social support and offering active support to others, social participation
Physical safety and security	one's home environment; work satisfaction; financial resources; health and social care (accessibility and quality); opportunities for acquiring new information and skills; participation in and opportunities for recreation/leisure activities; physical environment; and transport to health-care institutions
Spirituality	religion, and personal beliefs

According to the WHOQOL Group [23].

1.4 Conceptualizing QoL in CVDs

Determinants of HRQoL include the illness or disability itself as well as the type of medical intervention [18]. The main goal of any intervention in CVDs is to improve the patient's HRQoL by eliminating or reducing the influence of the disease. When constructing a HRQoL study, one should be mindful of whether the measurement is reflective of one patient or groups of patients, and whether the HRQoL measurement expresses a patient's status from the viewpoint of medical or social expectations.

Several dimensions are included in most studies examining HRQoL in CVDs. The first step is to define the physical, psychological, and social consequences of CVD, and to determine the influence of physical disability on changes to QoL. The second step is to identify individual reactions to disease-related dysfunctional states. Finally, the progress of rehabilitation is measured, with respect to minimizing psychosocial restrictions, and the effects of medical interventions and health education for the patient.

Studies examining HRQoL in CVDs should analyze a series of dimensions (Table 1.2).

Table 1.2 Health-Related Quality of Life in Cardiovascular Diseases

Dimensions	Indicators
Physical status	mobility, potential for self-care and independent everyday functioning
Emotional status	mood changes, anger, guilt, ambivalence, depressive symptoms, despair, preserving one's role as a patient, and expectations for the future
Social interactions	participation in different types of social activities, family relations, sexual activity, and marital satisfaction
Economic status	ability to ensure decent living conditions (i.e., standard of living), income, and employment
Intellectual status	memory, vigilance, ability to concentrate and learn
Perception of health status	self-rating of the severity of symptoms and degree of disability

Based on different studies [27 -32].

1.5 Future of QoL Studies

QoL studies will continue to develop dynamically despite conceptual difficulties or theoretical uncertainties. The focus of future studies should be to develop QoL models which may shed light on uncertainties connected with research. Future studies will probably be geared towards strengthening basic theoretical concepts and tailoring the definitions used to meet cultural requirements. One may also expect further development of the scales used to measure different dimensions of QoL. This will probably involve connecting the influence of disease and medical interventions with psychosocial determinants and resources from the period preceding changes in health status.

One may expect QoL to be universally applied in everyday clinical practice. It will begin to constitute the basic model for patient interaction and allow for a new quantification of therapeutic success, moving from a purely biological model to a more integrated bio–psycho–social model.

References

1. Bowling A (1995) Measuring disease: A review of disease-specific quality of life measurement scales. Open University Press Buckingham, Philadelphia
2. Bowling A (1995) What things are important in people's lives? A survey of the public's judgements to inform scales of health related quality of life. Soc Sci Med 41:1447-1462
3. Ebrahim S (1995) Clinical and public health perspectives and applications of health-related quality of life measurement. Soc Sci Med 41:1383-1394
4. Barofsky I (1986) Quality of life assessment. Evaluation of the concept. In: Ventafridda V, van Dam FSAM, Yancik r, Tamburini M (eds) Assessment of quality of life and cancer treatment. Elsevier, Amsterdam, pp 11-18
5. Frank RH (1989) Frames of reference and the quality of life. Quality of Life 79:80-88
6. Verbrugge L, Jette A (1994) The Disablement process. Soc Sci Med 38:1-14
7. Fava GA (1990) Methodological and Conceptual Issues in Research on Quality of Life. Psychother Psychosom 54:70-76
8. Pearlman RA, Uhlmann RF (1986) Perceptions of quality of life in elderly patients with cardiovascular disease. Quality of Life Cardiovasc Care 2:149-158
9. Davies O, Nutley SM, Mannion R (2000) Organisational culture and quality of health care. Qual Health Care 9:111-119
10. Noack H (1991) Conceptualizing and measuring health. In: Badura B, Kickbusch J (eds) Health Promotion Research Towards a New Social Epidemiology, vol 37. WHO, Copenhagen, pp 85-120
11. Fife B (1995) The measurement of meaning in illness. Soc Sci Med 40:1021-1028
12. Carr AJ (1996) A patient-centred approach to evaluation and treatment in rheumatoid arthritis: the development of a clinical tool to measure patient-perceived handicap. Br J Rheumatol 35:921-932
13. Anderson JP, Bush JW, Berry ChC (1986) Classifying function for health outcome and quality-of-life evaluation. Med Care 24:454-469
14. Higginson IJ, Carr AJ (2003) The clinical utility of quality of life measures. In: Carr AJ, Higginson IJ, Robinson P (eds) Quality of life. BMJ Books, BMA House, Tavistock Square, London pp 63-78
15. Bowling A (2002) Research methods in health. Investigating health and health services. Open University Press, Buckingham Philadelphia
16. WHOQOL Group (1995) The world health organisation quality of life assessment (WHOQOL): Position paper from the world health organisation. Soc Sci Med 41:1403-1409
17. Bowling A (2003) Current state of the art in quality of life measurement. In: Carr AJ, Higginson IJ, Robinson P (eds) Quality of life. BMJ Books, BMA House, Tavistock Square, London, pp 1-8
18. Brown N, Melville M, Gray D, Young T, MunroJ, Skene AM, Hampton JR (1999) Quality of life four years after acute myocardial infarction: short form 36 scores compared with a normal population. Heart 81:352-358
19. Arnold R, Ranchor AV, Sanderman R, Kempen GIJ, Ormel J, Suurmeijer TPBM (2004) The relative contribution of domains of quality of life to overall quality of life for different chronic diseases. Qual Life Res 13:883-896
20. Spilker B (1996) Introduction. In: Spilker B (ed) Quality of life and pharmacoeconomics in clinical trials. Second Edition. Lippincott-Raven Publishers, Philadelphia, pp 1-10
21. Siegrist J, Junge A (1989) Conceptual and methodological problems in research on the quality of life in clinical medicine. Soc Sci Med 29:463-468

22. McDowell I, Newell C (1996) Measuring Health. A Guide to Rating Scales and Questionnaires. Oxford University Press, New York-Oxford
23. Skevington SM (1999) Measuring quality of life in Britain: Introducing the WHOQOL-100. J Psychosom Res 47:449-459
24. Siegrist J, Siegrist K, Weber I (1986) Sociological concepts in the aetiology of chronic disease: the case of ischemic heart disease. Soc Sci Med 22: 247-253
25. Crocker Houde S, Devereaux Melillo K (2002) Cardiovascular health and physical activity in older adults: an integrative review of research methodology and results. Integrative Literature Reviews and Meta-Analyses. J Adv Nurs 38:219-234
26. Guillemin F, Bombardier C, Beaton D (1993) Cross-cultural adaptation of health-related quality of life measures literature review and proposed guidelines. J Clin Epidemiol 46:1417-1432
27. Graf J, Koch M, Dujardin R, Kersten A, Janssens U (2003) Health-related quality of life before, 1 month after, and 9 months after intensive care in medical cardiovascular and pulmonary patients. Crit Care Med 31:2163-2169
28. Bute BP, Mathew J, Blumenthal JA, Welsh-Bohmer K, White WD, Mark D, Landolfo K, Newman MF (2003) Female gender is associated with impaired quality of life 1 year after coronary artery bypass surgery. Psychosom Med 65:944-951
29. Lalonde L, O'Connor A, Joseph L, Grover SA (2004) Health-related quality of life in cardiac patients with dislipidemia and hypertension. Qual Life Res 13:793-804
30. Mena-Martin FJ, Martin-Escudero JC, Simal- Blanco F, Carretero-Ares JL, Arzua-Mouronte D, Herreros-Fernandez V (2003) Health–related quality of life of subjects with know and unknown hypertension: results from the population-based Hortega study. J Hypertens 21:1283-1289
31. Marmot M, Bartley M (2002) Social class and coronary heart disease. In: Stansfield S, Marmot M (eds) Stress and the heart – psychosocial pathways to coronary heart disease. BMJ Books, London, pp 5- 19
32. Jaarsveld CHM, Sanderman R, Ranchor AV, Ormel J, van Veldhuisen DJ, Kempen GIJM (2002) Gender-specific changes in quality of life following cardiovascular disease: A prospective study. J Clin Epidemiol 55:1105-1112

2 Quality of Life in Hypertensive Patients

Marek Klocek and Kalina Kawecka-Jaszcz

2.1 Introduction

The definition of health-related quality of life (HRQoL) includes the physical, psychological, and social aspects of positive wellbeing as well as the negative effects of illness, treatment, and infirmity. It refers to subjects' appraisals of their current level of functioning and satisfaction with it compared with what they perceive to be "ideal". HRQoL broadly encompasses those aspects of life which can influence or be influenced by "health". Usually HRQoL domains include physical, social and cognitive functioning as well as emotional wellbeing [1]. From a clinical perspective, after the manifestation and/or diagnosis of disease, this means that all of these dimensions may be influenced by the "health status" of the individual. Thus, this relationship is multidimensional. That is, good health is the result of biological, psychological, and social wellbeing; a disturbance in any of these areas (e.g., biological), results in disease, affects the other areas of wellbeing, and influences HRQoL.

Clinical studies are usually based on the effectiveness and practicality of a given treatment. These are most often based on "hard endpoints" such as survival, reduced morbidity, time-to-progression of disease, and prevalence of hospitalization. In the age of evidence-based medicine, "soft endpoints" (e.g., the wellbeing of the subject, capacity for everyday functioning and fulfillment of social roles, satisfaction with the state of health, physical activity, and mental efficiency) have less decisive roles. One reason for this situation is the difficulty associated with objectively measuring these categories. However, from the individuals' viewpoint, these aspects of health are probably most important, and often decide if and to what extent he or she complies with

M. Klocek (✉)
I Department of Cardiology and Hypertension
Jagiellonian University Medical College, Kraków, Poland
e-mail: marek.klocek@wp.pl

K. Kawecka-Jaszcz et al. (eds.), *Health-Related Quality of Life in Cardiovascular Patients*,
DOI: 10.1007/978-88-470-2769-5_2

the recommended treatment. Thus, HRQoL is a subjective concept that is dependent upon perception and individual preferences. Fortunately, soft endpoints: can be determined scientifically; are valid; are repeatable; and can provide suitable quantitative data.

In HRQoL studies, mild and/or moderate hypertension is considered to be the model for all asymptomatic or mildly symptomatic cardiovascular diseases (CVDs) requiring long-term treatment. In such diseases, treatment does not usually offer direct or immediate results that are experienced by the individual, yet should be continued to avoid the development of complications.

2.2 HRQoL as a Treatment Goal in Hypertension

Arterial hypertension is a major risk factor for CVD. Arterial hypertension is the leading cause of morbidity and mortality in modern societies, and is responsible for ≈13% of all deaths worldwide [2, 3]. In Poland, ≈9 million of the adult population (30%) have arterial hypertension but it is well-controlled (i.e., blood pressure (BP) < 140/90 mmHg) in only 26% of them [4]. The same situation is observed in other countries, with the exception of the USA and Canada [5, 6], where a higher percentage of subjects have well-controlled BP.

It is known that 20–40% of hypertensive subjects complain of: headaches; dizziness; fatigue; epistaxis; disturbances in mood and sleep; and/or sexual dysfunction. However, these symptoms are also frequently reported by subjects in the general population. Conversely, a large group of subjects (including those with systemic complications due to hypertension) may not notice any symptoms for many years [7, 8].

Well-designed clinical studies in large groups of subjects have confirmed that medicines currently used to decrease BP significantly increase longevity in hypertensive individuals even though various side effects (e.g., reduced wellbeing and/or psychomotor function) appear in the course of treatment. Impact of disease and treatment effects lead to changes in lifestyle that may also affect HRQoL and influence adherence to treatment, which can then be associated with poorly controlled BP in a population. It follows that ideal pharmacological therapy for hypertension should, in equal measure, prolong longevity as well as improve general wellbeing and functional status affected by the disease. Therefore, longevity and HRQoL are considered the two most sought-after and complementary goals of hypertension therapy.

2.3 Evaluating the HRQoL of Hypertensive Subjects

Most hypertensive subjects do not report any symptoms, so evaluating their HRQoL is a complex and multidimensional process. In this group, valuable data can be obtained on their emotional wellbeing, physical functioning, fulfillment of social roles, and other issues arising during treatment, as well as the way they perceive their own health. Health perception is an especially important factor influencing the decision to seek treatment and long-term compliance with treatment. A subject who perceives his/her health to be poor is more apt to seek medical care and more willing to comply with treatment.

Acceptance of a set definition of HRQoL is a requirement of any research project. Choosing an appropriate definition influences decisively what is to be measured in a given sample. Many authors feel that valuable medical studies on HRQoL should include the following categories:

- general wellbeing (feeling happy, satisfaction with life, positive and negative emotions, ability to relax);
- variables connected with physical health (physical activity, vitality, type and progression of symptoms of a given disease, health status, quality of sleep, sexual functioning);
- psychological variables (anxiety, depression, as well as cognitive, psychomotor, and intellectual function);
- everyday activities of the subject (work, rest, hobbies);
- social contact (family, friends, other social groups);
- external conditions (work, material situation, living conditions, social position).

Studies have shown that the best results with respect to HRQoL are obtained if the questionnaire containing various aspects of wellbeing is completed by the subject or by the spouse/partner [9]. The subjects' opinion should be considered the most important. One should never rely on the physician's opinion of HRQoL. A good example of this is a study from the 1980s by Jachuck et al. [10]. Hypertensive subjects, their physicians, and the closest relatives were asked in what way therapy influenced the HRQoL of subjects. The study demonstrated that stark differences existed between these three groups of respondents. All physicians felt that the HRQoL of their patients improved, whereas almost all relatives noted a declining QoL. Fifty percent of patients perceived their HRQoL to have improved and 50% of patients perceived their HRQoL to have worsened during antihypertensive treatment.

Generic and/or disease-specific measures can be used in HRQoL studies of hypertensive subjects. Generic instruments (e.g., Short Form Health Survey (SF-36), SF-12, Sickness Impact Profile (SIP), World Health Organization Quality of Life (WHO-QOL), EuroQoL-5D (EQ 5D)) are designed to be applicable across a wide range of populations and interventions. In contrast, disease-targeted measures (e.g., Subjective Symptoms Assessment Profile, Reitan Trail-making Test (TMT), Mini Mental State Examination) are designed to be relevant to a particular disease or selected health problem [11].

2.4 Factors Influencing the HRQoL of Hypertensive Subjects

Certain aspects of the relationship between high BP and HRQoL are unsolved. These include, in certain groups of subjects, the association with different domains and components of QoL as well as the influence of the: awareness of hypertension versus high BP; drug treatment in real conditions of use, control of BP on HRQoL.

Despite advances in knowledge, few HRQoL studies have taken place in large populations of subjects with arterial hypertension. Most studies focusing on hypertensive subjects describe the influence of antihypertensive drugs on various domains of HRQoL and, in many of these studies, the assessment of HRQoL was a secondary objective. Moreover, HRQoL is determined by several factors, and changes can seldom be explained by drug effects alone.

Most studies have shown a worse QoL of patients with hypertension than that of normotensive individuals. Population studies [12–14] have shown that the HRQoL of individuals who have not been treated as well as those who have been treated for arterial hypertension is lower by 10–20%, provided they are aware of their diagnosis. Similar results were shown in a study in Poland [15] of a population diagnosed with hypertension compared with normotensive subjects (Fig. 2.1).

HRQoL decreases with age for hypertensive and normotensive individuals [12]. However, for women with hypertension, deterioration in HRQoL occurs faster than for men. The reasons for a lowering of HRQoL in hypertensive subjects are complex. Some researchers argue that decreased HRQoL results directly from having a chronic disease: hypertension [16]. This argument is supported by reductions in HRQoL observed in subjects who are unaware of their disease as well as in diagnosed

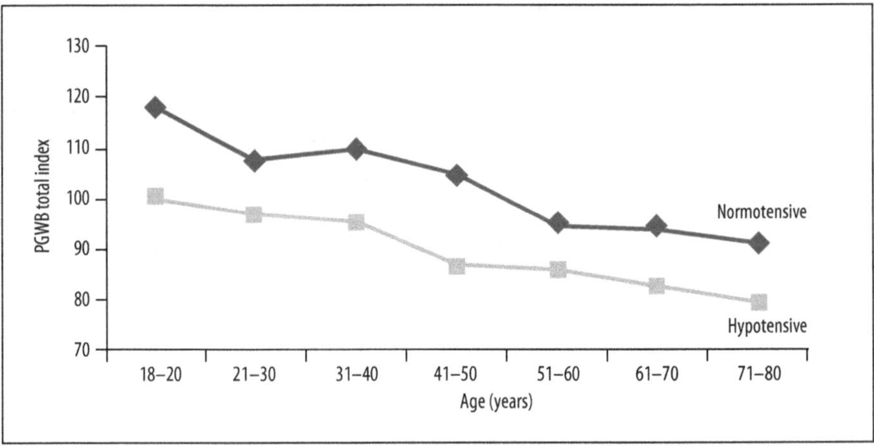

Fig. 2.1 Quality of Life measured with the Psychological General Wellbeing Index in hypertensive (n = 1539) and normotensive subjects (n = 995) according to age. Reproduced from [15], with permission

individuals before and after treatment commencement. Compared with normotensive individuals, subjects not treated by pharmacological means for hypertension may experience emotional disturbances, headaches and dizziness, sexual dysfunction, and are also characterized by inferior sleep quality and poor cognitive functioning [7]. These observations may or not be connected with elevated BP. Nevertheless, research has shown that better control over BP is associated with greater HRQoL, and that the participant is usually aware of the good control of BP and is pleased about it [17]. Individuals taking a placebo have reported similar symptoms to individuals being actively treated for hypertension. In addition, these same complaints are also noted in healthy individuals, whose HRQoL is higher.

For the reasons mentioned above, some researchers have suggested that a reduction in the HRQoL of subjects with hypertension may be because they were diagnosed with a disease (so-called "labeling effect"). Mena-Martin et al. [14] demonstrated that subjects who were aware of being hypertensive had a poorer QoL than those who were not aware. A reduction in HRQoL is further associated with anxiety, depression, worrying about one's health, physical functioning, absenteeism from work, and can even influence the lives of family members [18]. This effect – even before introducing pharmacotherapy – certainly reduces HRQoL in those diagnosed with hypertension [14]. Considering the risk of even further reductions in HRQoL, such patients require added attention during treatment. It was believed previously that the labeling effect had a significant role only in the early stages after the diagnosis. However, data showed that it may have a significant role for a few years, thereby negatively influencing an already declining HRQoL [19]. An already decreased HRQoL in untreated hypertensive individuals (as well as in individuals with undiagnosed hypertension) and the fact that individuals with chronic hypertension have a lower HRQoL than individuals with "white-coat hypertension" (which is diagnosed when BP is consistently > 140/90 mmHg in the office or clinical setting but is normal, < 135/85 mmHg, with ambulatory or home BP monitoring) [20], indicates that the labeling effect may not be the only factor influencing decreased HRQoL in hypertensive patients. Studies undertaken in Poland [15, 17] confirmed that, in complementary age groups, the general HRQoL of individuals being treated and not being treated by pharmacological means for hypertension was lower than that of the healthy population (Fig. 2.2). In this study, individuals aged < 40 years not yet treated for hypertension had a significantly greater HRQoL than subjects of the same age undergoing treatment (Fig. 2.2). Recently, Trevisol et al. found (in a population study of > 1,850 individuals; mean age, 47 years (men) and 52 years (women)) that HRQoL assessed with the SF-12 was worse in subjects with hypertension (in men and women) treated by pharmacological means when compared with untreated patients [21]. The lower HRQoL of hypertensive subjects was independent of age and education. Moreover, scores for women were lower than in men for all the SF-12 domains independent of the diagnosis of hypertension [22]. The findings of these studies suggest that a worse perception of wellbeing during treatment with antihypertensive drugs may cause problems with adherence to treatment in the future (especially in relatively young patients with a high HRQoL at baseline).

Conversely, data collected from multicenter studies suggest that untreated indi-

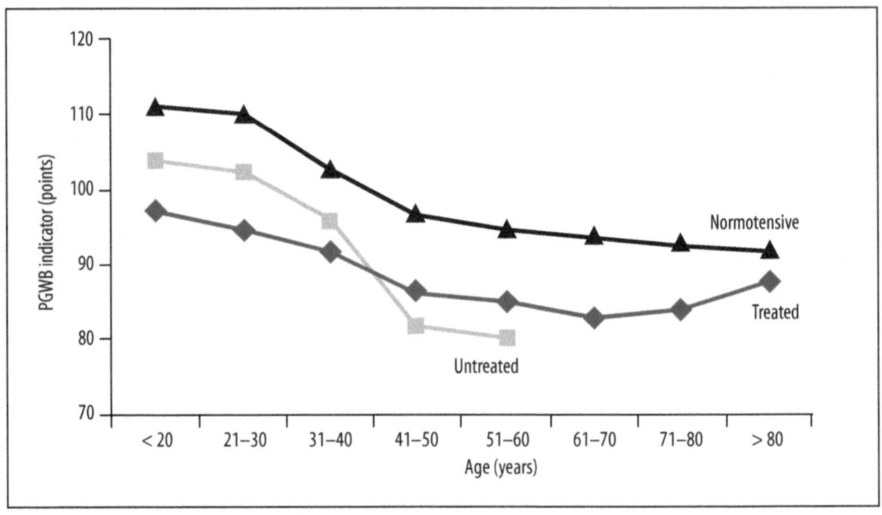

Fig. 2.2 Age-based comparison of Quality of Life (Psychological General Wellbeing Index) in treated (n = 1271) and untreated (n = 268) hypertensive subjects compared with normotensive controls (n = 995). Reproduced from [15], with permission

viduals may also have some degree of cognitive, psychomotor, and/or sensory dysfunction which may normalize after treatment. Thus, impaired HRQoL in hypertensive patients might be secondary to the awareness of hypertension, the adverse effects of drugs, or the presence of concomitant diseases, and not high BP *per se* [23].

The HRQoL of women with hypertension is lower than that in men of the same age [13, 15, 22]. Analogous differences between the sexes can also be observed in the general (healthy) population. However, the reasons for these differences are incompletely understood. In studies of hypertensive subjects in Poland [15, 17] decreases in the HRQoL of women during their fertile years were found to be attributed to reduced vitality and increased anxiety. During menopause, in addition to these two factors, reduced HRQoL was attributed to worsening health. In women aged > 60 years, HRQoL was affected by worsening health, amplified depression, and a feeling that "control was lost over their lives". These results were similar to those of other studies which examined significantly worsening HRQoL in older hypertensive women [13].

The Alameda County study was a 20-year follow-up study examining the psychosocial indicators of hypertension development [24]. With respect to the indicators present in men and women, the study found that, for men, stressors associated with work (e.g., low work status, unemployment, threat of unemployment) and for women, stressors associated with a poor psychological state (e.g., depression, loneliness, social isolation), were responsible for the development of hypertension. However, it is widely known that women, in general, present with more complaints concerning health than men, and are characterized by greater frustration, sleep problems, and excess housework, all of which can reduce their HRQoL.

Uncontrolled BP may be one of the most important factors influencing HRQoL. In some studies, an inverse relationship has been noted between higher systolic BP and diastolic BP and the level of HRQoL. This relationship was present across all age groups and applied to isolated systolic hypertension in elderly individuals. It has also been suggested that increased diastolic BP > 95 mmHg is associated with worse wellbeing, and that intensive antihypertensive therapy decreases the frequency and progression of side effects [25]. Results from the Trial of Antihypertensive Interventions and Management (TAIM) also found that reducing BP, irrespective of the treatment option, led to improved quality of sleep, increased sexual activity, and satisfaction with the state of one's health [26]. However, the results of the Treatment of Mild Hypertension Study (TOMHS) [27] suggested that, even with a reduction in BP, differences existed in the influence of specific groups of drugs on HRQoL.

Taking into account current evidence, it is difficult to state if the impact of antihypertensive treatment on HRQoL is dependent solely upon a reduction in BP or is possibly due to the effect of certain drugs. It is worth noting that, though BP was responsible for only 17% of the variability in general HRQoL in one of our studies, it was the strongest clinical factor connected with HRQoL [17].

It is also known that HRQoL changes with the number of drugs used. Based on available data, it seems that the HRQoL of hypertensive subjects is associated (i) with the degree of BP control and (ii) with the number of drugs used. These results confirm conclusions reached in clinical studies undertaken in recent years [13, 28] concerning the necessity for good control of BP (BP < 140/90 mmHg), including its potential influence on improving HRQoL.

Education is one of the most important factors determining HRQoL. Normotensive and hypertensive individuals with higher levels of education, irrespective of sex, are characterized by a higher HRQoL. In contrast, low levels of education and low socioeconomic status are associated with greater morbidity and mortality due to hypertension as well as a reduced HRQoL [13, 27, 29]. These individuals often constitute a subpopulation not very compliant with therapy, who care less about their health and – as shown by epidemiological studies – belong to a group at higher risk of developing cardiovascular complications.

Obesity is another important factor influencing HRQoL, especially in hypertensive women. In women, obesity negatively influences such dimensions of HRQoL as physical health, quality of sleep, sexuality, capacity for everyday functioning, and social interactions.

Side effects of drugs constitute an important problem in the pharmacotherapy of arterial hypertension. It has been argued that they may explain the poor effectiveness of antihypertensive therapy observed in everyday practice. Some of the side effects are non-specific (e.g., headaches), whereas other side effects result from the class of drugs used (e.g., coughing in those treated with angiotensin-converting enzyme inhibitors (ACEIs) or facial flushing and peripheral edema in subjects treated with calcium-channel blockers). In a study undertaken in Poland [30] only one-quarter of those treated with antihypertensive drugs directly complained to physicians about side effects, whereas > 70% of them experienced various symptoms (e.g., dry mouth, polyuria, dry cough).

A useful indicator of QoL is the number of drugs taken by the subject. A close relationship exists between the number of drugs taken and HRQoL. It is known that, to reach BP control, > 60% of patients must take 2–3 drugs. Hence, in keeping with guidelines set by the European Society of Hypertension, we recommended combination preparations. These are characterized not only by their effectiveness but also by a reduced frequency of side effects due to their decreased dosage,.

A study carried out in Poland in a population with essential arterial hypertension [15, 17] demonstrated that sociodemographic factors such as age, sex, education, and family burden accounted for ≈36% of the general QoL. In addition, various clinical factors also influence HRQoL (e.g., BP, effectiveness of BP control, disease complications, number of drugs used, body weight). In hypertensive subjects, these clinical factors explained a further 37% of the variability in HRQoL (Fig. 2.3). This observation further supports the view that HRQoL is determined by various factors, and that no factor can be considered to be separate from the others, nor discounted in any

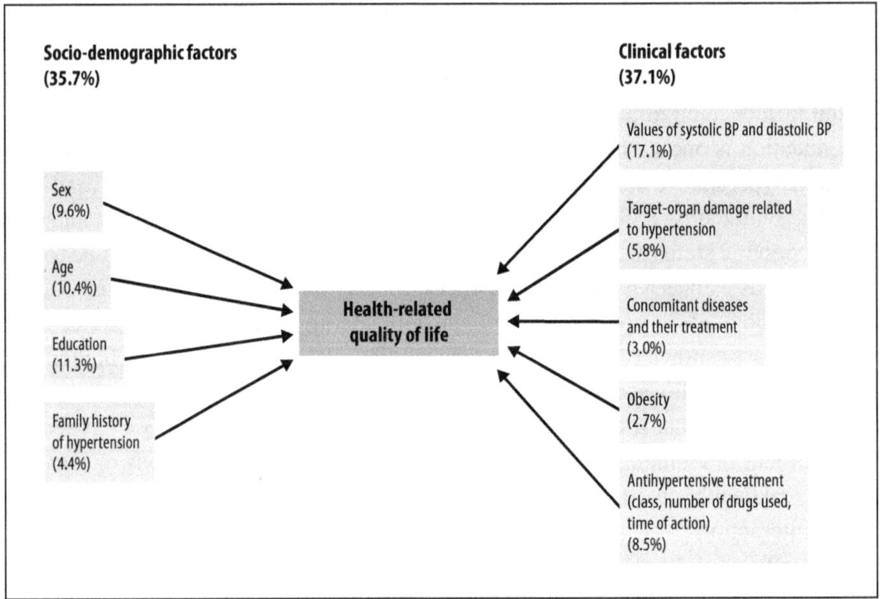

Fig. 2.3 Socio-demographic and clinical factors influencing health-related Quality of Life in hypertension subjects. Reproduced from [17], with permission

way. Furthermore, a common methodological and interpretative mistake which should be avoided is studying only one factor influencing HRQoL.

The data shown above suggest that improving the HRQoL of hypertensive individuals is dependent upon many factors. Considering the relationship between elevated BP and degree of cardiovascular risk, the first step is BP control. Analyses of data from a subpopulation of 922 subjects from the Hypertension Optimal Treatment Study found that reducing diastolic pressure to < 80 mmHg was safe and could lead to significant improvement in general wellbeing [28]. This effect was noted during use of a long-acting calcium antagonist.

A study performed in Poland [17] found the highest HRQoL level, both in hypertensive men and women when systolic BP was 125-140 mmHg and diastolic BP was 75 90 mmHg. Prospective studies confirmed that a reduction in systolic BP and diastolic BP slowed down the process of decreasing HRQoL in older age, and positively influenced psychological (e.g., cognitive function, mood) and physical (e.g., physical dexterity, vitality) ability. The Systolic Hypertension in Europe (Syst-Eur) Trial was devoted to the treatment of isolated systolic hypertension in the elderly. The results from this study suggested the possibility for decreasing the frequency of dementia using calcium antagonists [31]. Data from this study also suggested that lowering BP leads to improved sleep quality, a lower prevalence of somatic complaints, increased satisfaction with one's health, and improved sexual function.

It is equally important to treat other risk factors for CVD. In non-pharmacological management, reducing the weight of the subject seems to exert the greatest effect on HRQoL. Some studies, including the TOMHS, confirm this point: reducing weight improved HRQoL not only during antihypertensive treatment but also with a placebo. It is known that normalizing BP using non-pharmacological methods increases HRQoL more so than by pharmacological treatment alone [27].

Data suggest that regular physical activity, reducing the consumption of alcohol, and stopping smoking may slightly improve HRQoL. Restricting sodium intake has not yet been definitively proven to increase QoL. HRQoL has also been shown to be positively influenced by certain relaxation techniques used to lower BP. However, application of such techniques requires time, skilled personnel, and cooperation from the patient. When beginning lifestyle modification, a slight worsening in HRQoL should be expected initially (especially if incorporating many lifestyle changes simultaneously). Afterwards, HRQoL improves significantly.

2.4 QoL and Antihypertensive Treatment

It has been found that significant decreases in HRQoL, even before starting treatment, are associated with an increased risk of death from CVD independent of classical risk factors (including an increased risk of stroke) [32].

The vast majority of clinical studies examining the HRQoL of hypertensive subjects have focused on monotherapy. Simultaneously, new research programs encompassing thousands of subjects showed that combined therapy (i.e., two or three drugs) should be used in > 60% of individuals with hypertension to achieve appropriate control of BP. Theoretically, combined therapy should change HRQoL but in a manner that is dependent upon the specific drugs chosen. Choice of drug is of fundamental importance from the perspective of the HRQoL of the subject. Despite methodological differences between studies, results suggest that significant qualitative and quantitative differences influence the effect of the main antihypertensive drugs upon HRQoL. It has also been suggested that differences exist between the drugs in each group. The time of action of the drug is of significant importance to HRQoL: longer-acting drugs are more positively rated by patients than short-acting drugs. Of equal importance is the dosage: in general, the lower the dose of an antihypertensive drug, the higher the HRQoL of the individual. This is why combining a small and medium dose of two drugs in one tablet is especially advantageous. New-generation drugs are better for HRQoL than older-generation agents. Therefore, careful attention should be paid to the choice of drugs used in clinical practice. Long-acting drugs (especially ones which are used once daily and offer minimal and/or infrequent side effects) should be recommended (Table 2.1). The values of BP that are optimal for HRQoL are 130–140 mmHg for systolic BP and 75–90 mmHg for diastolic BP [15, 28].

2.5 Lifestyle Modification

Large studies examining the influence on HRQoL of non-pharmacological management of arterial hypertension are lacking. Single studies carried out many years ago have confirmed that subjects who have been able to reduce their BP without drugs have a better HRQoL than individuals being treated by pharmacological means. In particular, reducing body weight influences improvement in HRQoL [28]. However, restricting the amount of sodium in the diet may exacerbate erectile dysfunction and lead to fatigue and disturbed sleep.

Instituting changes in the lifestyle of subjects interferes with their already accepted behaviors, which not necessarily influences their HRQoL in a positive way. These recommendations exert a psychological effect on some individuals who consider themselves to be "restricted" and "pressured" into reorganizing their lives to accommodate new dietary requirements or to incorporate regular physical activity. Such individuals experience a temporary decline in their wellbeing, for example, due to physiologic effects after ceasing smoking or restricting alcohol consumption. They may also lose some of their social privileges due to the effect of changing their current lifestyle. This period of worsening HRQoL experienced after lifestyle modification may last from 3

Table 2.1 Common side effects of antihypertensive drugs

Drug class	Side effects	Psychomotor function
High blood pressure alone	Headache, epistaxis, blurred vision, palpitations, tiredness	
Diuretics		
Thiazide	Impotence, decreased libido, lethargy, constipation, nausea, dizziness	
Indapamide	Dizziness, constipation, rarely decreases libido	Improved verbal and intellectual function
Beta-adrenolytics	Shortness of breath, lethargy, dizziness, vivid dreaming, cold extremities, vision problems, decreased tolerance for physical activity	Prolonged complex-reaction time, impaired verbal memory and psychosensory function, depression
Calcium antagonists		
Dihydropyridines	Headaches and dizziness, hot flushes, erythema, lower-limb edema, nausea	Improved short-term memory, improved psychophysical vitality, delayed development of dementia?
Non-dihydropyridines	Constipation, headaches and dizziness, nausea	
Angiotensin-converting enzyme inhibitors	Dry cough, rash, trouble with or lack of taste	Opioid-resistant action, improved memory?
Angiotensin II-receptor blockers	Incidence of side effects similar to placebo – most often headaches and dizziness	Improved memory and learning ability? Delayed development of dementia?
Alpha-blockers	Orthostatic hypotension, fatigue, lethargy, headaches, nasal sinus edema	
Centrally acting drugs		
Rilmenidine, moxonidine	Minimal lethargy	
Methyldopa	Diarrhea, fatigue, weakness, dry mouth, vivid dreams	Worsened verbal memory
Clonidine	Fatigue, sleep disturbance, dry mouth, constipation, lethargy, sedation	Prolonged complex-reaction time Depression – especially with reserpine

months to 6 months. This is a critical period in which the subject often gives up instituting lifestyle changes. This is why he/she should be under supervision during this time and supported in his/her efforts to maintain the necessary changes in lifestyle.

2.6 Drugs Used to Treat Hypertension

2.6.1 Diuretics

The ways in which diuretics influence HRQoL has not been documented fully. Studies have confirmed that individuals being treated with diuretics more often complain about sexual dysfunction, depressed mood, and/or cognitive dysfunction (Table 1). The negative influence of thiazide diuretics on sexual function has been confirmed in multicenter studies such the Medical Research Council (MRC) study and TAIM study [26], in which 11–25% (chlortalidone) and 18% (bendroflumethiazide, hydrochlorothiazide) of treated male subjects noted an increased prevalence of impotence. Conversely, only 1.6% more males using spironolactone noted an increased prevalence of impotence compared with the placebo group. In the TOMHS [33], after 24 months, the prevalence of impotence in the group treated with chlorthalidone was 17% and was 8% in the placebo group ($p < 0.03$). However, after 48 months of observation, no difference in the prevalence of impotence was noted between the two groups.

Paran et al. [34] noted a significant improvement in certain dimensions of the HRQoL of hypertensive subjects 6–9 months after withdrawing thiazide diuretics. However, after withdrawing diuretics, participants did not reach the same level of HRQoL as patients who were never previously treated with diuretics. Compared with thiazide diuretics, the non-thiazide diuretic indapamide was found to be tolerated just as well by younger patients as those aged > 65 years and caused: fewer side effects; fewer sleep disturbances; a decreased prevalence of impotence [35].

Diuretics such as chlorthalidone and especially hydrochlorothiazide used in large doses exert a decisively negative influence on HRQoL. Lower doses of these drugs as well as spironolactone have a better influence on HRQoL. For HRQoL, in keeping with current recommendations, diuretics should be used in small doses, and often do not yield any side effects.

2.6.2 Beta-adrenergic Receptor Blockers

The influence of beta-blockers on HRQoL is focused on the typical side effects and symptoms these drugs may evoke in the central nervous system (CNS) (Table 1). These symptoms arise from the lipophilic property of certain beta-blockers, which allows them to readily penetrate the blood–brain barrier. CNS-related side effects elicited by beta-blockers most often include: disturbed phases of sleep; insomnia; colorful and vivid dreams; nightmares; memory problems; hallucinations; a feeling of psychophysical fatigue; and emotional instability. In some subjects, low moods and depression may be present several months after beginning treatment with beta-blockers.

However, the minimally anxiolytic action of beta-blockers must be noted, and is especially pronounced in the elderly.

One of the most often discussed problems connected with the use of beta-blockers is their influence on the sexual health of hypertensive individuals. The TAIM study [26] did not find differences between the sexual function of men and women treated with atenolol and the placebo group. Similarly, in the 4-year TOMHS [33], the influence of acebutolol on the sexual function of hypertensive subjects was similar to that of the placebo group. In the TOMHS, the frequency of erectile dysfunction recorded at the start of the study (before beginning treatment) was strongly correlated with systolic BP. Men with systolic BP > 140 mmHg noted a frequency of erectile dysfunction that was twofold greater than that of men with lower systolic BP. These observations point to a direct influence of BP on the development of sexual dysfunction in men. Sexual dysfunction may appear as a result of using certain antihypertensive drugs, and constitutes an important cause of non-compliance by subjects. The negative influence of beta-blockers (especially non-selective) on the sexual function of men being treated for hypertension has long been reported. Current data do not provide similar observations on the new generation of beta-blockers [36].

Certain beta-blockers, such as bisoprolol, influence HRQoL more positively than enalapril. Bisoprolol also boasts a more positive influence on HRQoL when compared with Adalat retard (nifedipine) [37]. However, a direct comparison of two beta-blockers, atenolol and bisoprolol, did not find that one influenced HRQoL more than the other.

Atenolol and metoprolol (including the extended-release form) are the drugs most often used in studies on the HRQoL of individuals treated with beta-blockers. Both drugs similarly influence HRQoL if used in comparative doses. In clinical studies they are used as a reference point to gauge the influence of a new drug on QoL. It seems that the results of several HRQoL studies using atenolol can be extended to most other beta-blockers with the exception of propranolol, the profile of which is decidedly worse (though some recent studies are beginning to express a more positive opinion of this drug). Limited observations are also giving hope to a newer generation of drugs such as carvedilol, celiprolol, betaxolol, and nebivolol.

2.6.3 Calcium Antagonists

With respect to HRQoL, amlodipine is one of the best-rated calcium antagonists (Table 2.1). Omvik et al. [38] studied the tolerance, effectiveness, and influence of amlodipine on HRQoL compared with enalapril. This study found that both drugs yielded a similar effect of reducing BP, whereas an improved HRQoL was noted in those using amlodipine. This study continued to be carried out in an open phase for 2 years [39] with patients who, using amlodipine, achieved BP control in the first year of treatment.

During those 2 years, the ability of amlodipine to decrease BP was maintained and a minimal (though statistically significant: 2–4%) improvement in HRQoL parameters was also observed.

In another multicenter, double-blind, randomized study comparing amlodipine and enalapril, two questionnaires were incorporated to measure general and specific HRQoL [40]. Both drugs reduced BP to a similar extent after 8 weeks, but a significant improvement in HRQoL was noted only in those treated with amlodipine, an effect especially noticeable in patients aged > 50 years. This improvement in the HRQoL of subjects using only amlodipine was associated with reduced anxiety, a reduced level of depressed mood, and improved general wellbeing and vitality.

A similar study was conducted by Weir et al. It compared the effect of amlodipine, bisoprolol, or enalapril monotherapy on the HRQoL of individuals with mild and moderate hypertension. Improvement in general HRQoL and hypertension-related QoL was confirmed in those using amlodipine and bisoprolol, but not enalapril [41].

Leonetti et al. [42] compared the use of lacidipine and lercanidipine (lipophilic calcium antagonists) with amlodipine for their side effects and influence on the wellbeing of hypertensive subjects. These individuals noted better tolerance to treatment based on lacidipine and lercanidipine than that based on amlodipine.

Isradipine, if used by older women, improved HRQoL (i.e., wellbeing, physical and emotional state, cognitive function, fulfilling social roles) to a similar extent as that seen with atenolol and enalapril, but subjects reported significantly fewer side effects than with atenolol and enalapril. In the Lomir (isradipine) Multicenter Study in Israel (LOMIR-MCT-IL) [43], 3 months of monotherapy using isradipine was found to improve HRQoL and semantic memory. It was again confirmed that the HRQoL of hypertensive subjects was lower than the HRQoL of normotensive individuals.

Felodipine was the drug of choice in the Hypertension Optimal Treatment (HOT) study, which was the first to confirm that the extent to which HRQoL improves is dependent upon how intensively BP is lowered [28]. In the HOT study, the highest HRQoL was noted for subjects whose diastolic BP was lowered to ≈81 mmHg. Participants were aware of their "good" BP. It was also demonstrated that, in most patients, normalizing BP requires a combination regimen of two or three drugs. The positive influence of felodipine on HRQoL was also noted in other studies.

The Syst-Eur study demonstrated that using nitrendipine as an active treatment for isolated systolic hypertension in subjects aged > 60 years led to a significant (42%) reduction in mortality due to stroke and a 26% reduction in mortality due to cardiovascular events [44]. Not long after, it was demonstrated that active treatment diminished the risk of developing dementia in this group of individuals [31]. The results of an analysis comparing the influence of active treatment and placebo on HRQoL in subjects with isolated systolic hypertension were unexpected [45]. The Syst-Eur study used a set of questionnaires to examine different dimensions of HRQoL: the Brief Assessment Index (to measure depression and mood disorders), TMT A and B (to measure cognitive function), and the SIP (to measure general QoL). Complete data concerning HRQoL was received from 610 subjects, with an observation period of 4 years. After data analyses, individuals treated actively with nitrendipine had worse TMT results (cognitive dysfunction) and complained of more social-interaction problems than subjects in the placebo group. No differences were noted between active treatment and placebo in terms of changes in mood, depression, or other SIP subscales. The authors concluded that active treatment in the Syst-Eur study was associated with a minimally detrimental affect on the HRQoL in individuals with isolated systolic hypertension [45].

An interesting analysis of the Syst-Eur study published in 2002 detailed some of the reasons for withdrawing participants from the study. Those data found that subjects treated actively for hypertension were tenfold less likely to be withdrawn from the study due to uncontrolled hypertension. Conversely, that group was also tenfold more likely to experience side effects typical of nitrendipine (i.e., ankle edema, flushing). Finally, active treatment using nitrendipine or a combination of nitrendipine and enalapril was cited twice as often to be a reason for withdrawal from the study than using a placebo. Despite better control of BP, subjects being treated actively were more likely to experience side effects, and 15–20% cited this as a reason for withdrawing from the study. These effects are probably responsible for the decrease in HRQoL of subjects participating in the Syst-Eur study mentioned above [46].

2.6.4 Angiotensin-Converting Enzyme Inhibitors (ACEIs)

In 1986, Croog et al. [47] published a double-blind study on the QoL of 540 subjects with mild and moderate hypertension chosen from a randomized and multicultural sample using a standardized questionnaire: the Psychological General Wellbeing Index (PGWB). Participants using captopril monotherapy reported a minimal (though significant) increase in their wellbeing, ability to work, and cognitive function. However, adding a diuretic to any one of the three drugs used in the study (captopril, propranolol, methyldopa) yielded a negative affect on HRQoL, but addition of a diuretic was in response to poor control of BP.

Subsequent HRQoL studies confirmed a more beneficial profile of captopril compared with that of propranolol, as well as those of the short-acting agents nifedipine and verapamil. In many studies, captopril and enalapril are considered to be "baseline drugs" to which newer ACEIs as well as other antihypertensive drugs are compared in HRQoL studies (Table 2.1).

In a face-to-face study of 379 subjects, Testa et al. [48] compared the influence of captopril and enalapril on HRQoL: they found this influence to be dependent upon the initial level of HRQoL. If at baseline patients reported a reduced QoL, neither captopril nor enalapril lead to further reductions; instead, they may even lead to improvement in, for example, vitality and emotional control. Conversely, in individuals with high HRQoL (i.e., those not experiencing any subjective symptoms of hypertension), reduced HRQoL was noted after treatment with enalapril, but not after captopril. These results have been the topic of many discussions and editorials concerning the treatment of asymptomatic patients, and mainly reflect the phenomenon of "regression to the mean".

When analyzing the influence of enalapril and atenolol on cognitive functions, enalapril had a more positive influence on memory, reaction time, physical coordination, and concentration. In light of current knowledge comparing the influence of ACEIs on HRQoL, captopril is at an advantage against propranolol and methyldopa, as is enalapril against atenolol, but not against bisoprolol.

The newer ACEI cilazapril was found to be more effective in lowering BP than nifedipine (including having a decisively better influence on certain aspects of the HRQoL of hypertensive individuals), whereas both drugs did not influence the memory or learning ability of subjects. Compared to metoprolol, using lisinopril improved the job activity of hypertensive patients and, compared to nifedipine, less side effects were noticed which could negatively impact HRQoL and as compared to atenolol improvement in sexual function in hypertensive males was found [49].

From the perspective of HRQoL, ACEIs such as cilazapril, lisinopril, perindopril, chinapril, ramipril, and trandolapril have been recognized for their positive effects. However, studies with large cohorts of hypertensive subjects taking these drugs are lacking. ACEIs, followed by new-generation calcium antagonists, yield the most positive effect on HRQoL. Some authors argue that, because of the small number of side effects, ACEIs have a generally better profile for their overall influence on HRQoL when compared with calcium antagonists.

2.6.5 Angiotensin II-Receptor Antagonists

It is widely known that angiotensin II-receptor antagonists are characterized by very few side effects, even when compared with a placebo (Table 2.1). This class of drug is the most readily accepted by patients in the treatment of chronic hypertension [50]. In the Losartan Versus Amlodipine (LOA) study [51] (which was a double-blind trial), 898 hypertensive subjects were treated for 12 weeks to evaluate the influence of losartan and amlodipine on HRQoL. Though both drugs yielded a similar effect with respect to tolerance and lowering BP, HRQoL was improved only in the group treated with losartan; it remained unchanged in the amlodipine group. In another study comparing the HRQoL of those treated with losartan or nifedipine gastrointestinal therapeutic system (GITS), nifedipine was at a decisive disadvantage. It has also been shown that losartan improves QoL and cognitive function in the elderly.

Eprosartan yielded a minimally more negative influence on the HRQoL of hypertensive subjects when compared with enalapril, even though enalapril more often caused coughing. A subsequent study did not find differences in the HRQoL of hypertensive subjects treated with either drug. Conversely, valsartan, compared with enalapril, yielded a significantly more positive influence on the cognitive function of hypertensive subjects [52]. Other studies of men treated with valsartan monotherapy suggested, compared with the beta-blockers carvedilol and atenolol, a significant improvement in sexual function, even with an antihypertensive effect similar to that seen with other drugs. Valsartan also yields a positive influence on the sexual function of hypertensive women [53].

During treatment with an 80-mg daily dose of telmisartan, a significant improvement in HRQoL measured using the PGWB was observed in younger age groups as well as in those aged > 65 years in men and women [54]. A considerable improvement in HRQoL was achieved in subjects whose BP stabilized during the course of the study. Telmisartan was also shown to be more effective than atenolol in its positive influence upon HRQoL.

Recently, new data from a non-interventional short-term study have been published [55]. In that trial, > 4,200 hypertensive subjects treated in primary care were involved; they then had additional treatment with olmesartan or were switched to olmesartan therapy. After 6 weeks of treatment, HRQoL improved as measured by the SF-12 questionnaire.

New data from the Trial of Preventing Hypertension (TROPHY) study has provided evidence that treatment with candesartan compared with placebo in individuals with prehypertension and a relatively high baseline HRQoL leads to maintenance of a high level of HRQoL during a four-year observation period [56].

2.6.6 Centrally Acting Drugs and Alpha-Adrenergic Receptor Blockers

In a study in which subjects with hypertension and diabetes mellitus used older centrally acting drugs (clonidine or methyldopa) in monotherapy, 80% of men reported an improvement in sexual function once these drugs were switched to the alpha-adrenergic receptor blocker prazosine. In the TOMHS [33], the lowest prevalence of erectile dysfunction, similar to that in the placebo group, was noted in those treated with the newer alpha-adrenergic receptor blocker doxazosine. Men who reported erectile dysfunction at baseline observed improvement after treatment with only one of the TOMHS drugs: doxazosine. It has been shown that doxazosine improves HRQoL especially in men with prostatic hypertrophy being treated for hypertension [57].

Older-generation centrally acting drugs seem to rank worse against newer-generation drugs (Table 1). This is because of several problematic side effects manifested during treatment (e.g., depressed mood, sleep disturbances, trouble with verbal memory, fatigue). Reserpine, which is used very rarely, also negatively affects the HRQoL of hypertensive individuals.

The new-generation drugs rilmenidine and moxonidine act by modulating the function of imidazole receptors. They have been a significant breakthrough in the evaluation of the influence of centrally acting drugs on HRQoL. Rilmenidine in monotherapy positively influences wellbeing and psychomotor function without the sedative effect of older-generation drugs. Moxonidine can also improve the sexual function of subjects with hypertension, and tolerance to this drug is comparable with that of placebo [58]. However, studies with large groups of patients are required to determine the influence of new-generation, centrally acting drugs on HRQoL.

2.7 Conclusions

In the last two decades, almost every new antihypertensive drug has been evaluated for its influence on different aspects of HRQoL. This allows for easier decision-making in clinical practice. The development of more effective and safer drugs that are better suited to the problems of patients can be helped by developing an appreciation of the widely understood concepts of wellbeing and patient functioning. One should have an understanding of the multidimensional effects of hypertension as a disease, the effects of other risk factors for CVD, and the pharmacological treatment of hypertension.

References

1. Osoba D (2005) Health-related quality of life outcomes in clinical trials. In: Fayers P, Hays R (eds.) Assessing quality of life in clinical trials. Methods and practice. Oxford University Press, New York, pp 259-274
2. Kearney PM, Whelton M, Reynolds K et al (2004) Worldwide prevalence of hypertension: a systematic review. J Hypertens 22:11-19
3. Pereira M, Lunet N, Azevedo A et al (2009) Differences in prevalence, awareness, treatment and control of hypertension between developing and developed countries. J Hypertens 27:963-975
4. Zdrojewski T, Szpakowski P, Bandosz P et al (2004) Arterial hypertension in Poland in 2002. J Hum Hypertens 18:557-562
5. Egan BM, Zhao Y, Axon RN (2010) US trends in prevalence, awareness, treatment and control of hypertension, 1988-2008. JAMA 303:2043-2050
6. Campbel NR, Khan NA, Hill MD et al (2009) 2009 Canadian Hypertension Education Program recommendations: the scientific summary – an annual update. Can J Cardiol 25:271-277
7. Wiklund IK (1996) Hypertension. In: Spilker B (ed) Quality of Life and Pharmacoeconomics in Clinical Trials. Lippincott-Raven Publishers, Philadelphia, pp 893-902
8. Coyne KS, Davis D, Frech F et al (2002) Health-related quality of life in patients treated for hypertension: a review of the literature from 1990-2000. Clin Ther 24:142-169
9. Addington-Hall J, Kalra L (2001) Who should measure quality of life? BMJ 322:1417-1420
10. Jachuck SJ, Brierly H, Jachuck S et al (1982) The effect of hypotensive drugs on the quality of life. J R Coll Gen Pract 32:103-105

11. Hays RD (2005) Generic versus disease-targeted instruments. In: Fayers P, Hays R (eds.) Assessing quality of life in clinical trials. Methods and practice. Oxford University Press, New York, pp 3-8
12. Bardage C, Isacson DGL (2001) Hypertension and health-related quality of life: an epidemiological study in Sweden. J Clin Epidemiol 54:172-181
13. Roca-Cusachs A, Dalfo A, Badia X et al (2001) Relation between clinical and therapeutic variables and quality of life in hypertension. J Hypertens 19:1913-1919
14. Mena-Martin FJ, Martin-Escudero JC, Simal-Blanco F et al (2003) Health-related quality of life of subjects with known and unknown hypertension: results from the population-based Hortega study. J Hypertens 21:1283-1289
15. Klocek M, Kawecka-Jaszcz K (2003) Quality of life in patients with arterial hypertension. Part I: The effect of socio-demographic factors. Przegl Lek 60:92-100
16. Erickson SR, Williams BC, Gruppen LD (2001) Perceived symptoms and health-related quality of life reported by uncomplicated hypertensive patients compared to normal controls. J Hum Hypertens 15:539-548
17. Klocek M, Kawecka-Jaszcz K (2003) Quality of life in patients with arterial hypertension. Part I: The effect of clinical factors. Przegl Lek 60:101-106
18. Battersby C, Hartlery K, Fletcher AE (1995) Quality of life in treated hypertension: a case-control community based study. J Hum Hypertens 9:854-859
19. Mold JW, Hamm RM, Jafri B (2000) The effect of labeling on perceived ability to recover from acute illnesses and injures. J Fam Pract 49:437-440
20. Coelho R, Santos A, Ribeiro L et al (1999) Differences in behavior profile between normotensive subject and patients with white-coat and sustained hypertension. J Psychosom Res 46:15-27
21. Trevisol DJ, Moreira LB, Fuchs FD et al (2011) Health-related quality of life is worse in individuals with hypertension under drug treatment: results of population-based study. J Hum Hypertens 26:374-380
22. Trevisol DJ, Moreira LB, Kerkhoff A et al (2011) Health-related quality of life and hypertension: a systematic review and meta-analysis of observational studies. J Hypertens 29:179-188
23. Korhonen PE, Kivelä SL, Kautiainen H et al (2011) Health-related quality of life and awareness of hypertension. J Hypertens 29:2070-2074
24. Levenstein S, Smith MW, Kaplan GA (2001) Psychosocial predictors of hypertension in men and women. Arch Intern Med 161:1341-1346
25. Hansson L for the BBB Study Group (1994) The BBB Study: the effect of intensified antihypertensive treatment on the level of blood pressure, side-effects, morbidity and mortality in "well-treated" hypertensive patients. Blood Pres 3:248-254
26. Wassertheil-Smoller S, Blaufox MD, Oberman A et al (1991) Effect of antihypertensives on sexual function and quality of life: the TAIM Study. An Intern Med 114:613-620
27. Grimm RH, Grandits GA, Cutler JA et al (1997) Relationships of quality-of-life measures to long-term lifestyle and drug treatment in the Treatment of Mild Hypertension Study (TOMHS). Arch Intern Med 157:638-648
28. Wilkund IK, Halling K, Ryden-Bergsten T et al (1997) Does lowering the blood pressure improve the mood? Quality-of-life results from the Hypertension Optimal Treatment (HOT) Study. Blood Pres 6:357-364
29. Tedesco MA, Di Salvo G, Caputo S (2001) Educational level and hypertension: how socioeconomic differences condition health care. J Hum Hypertens 15:727-731
30. Pająk A, Klocek M, Grodzicki T et al (1999) Adverse symptoms and effectiveness of treatment of essential arterial hypertension. Nadciśnienie Tętnicze 3:182-191
31. Forette F, Seux ML, Staessen JA et al (1998) Prevention of dementia in randomised double-blind placebo-controlled Systolic Hypertension in Europe (Syst-Eur) trial. Lancet 352:1347-1351
32. Agewall S, Wilkstrand J, Fagerberg B (1998) Stroke was predicted by dimensions of quality of life in treated hypertensive men. Stroke 29:2329-2333

33. Grimm RH, Grandits GA, Prineas RJ et al (1997) Long-term effects on sexual function of five antihypertensive drugs and nutritional hygienic treatment in hypertensive men and women: Treatment of Mild Hypertension Study (TOMHS). Hypertension 29:8-14
34. Paran E, Anson O, Neumann L (1996) The effects of diuretics on quality of life of hypertensive patients. J Hum Hypertens 10:147-152
35. Guez D, Crocq L, Sefavian A et al (1988) Effects of indapamide on the quality of life of hypertensive patients. Am J Med 84:53-58
36. Van Bortel LM, Bulpitt CJ, Fici F (2005) Quality of life and antihypertensive effect with nebivolol and losartan. Am J Hypertens 18:1060-1066
37. Bulpitt CJ, Connor M, Schulte M et al (2000) Bisoprolol and nifedipine retard in elderly hypertensive patients: effect on quality of life. J Hum Hypertens 14:205-212
38. Omvik P, Thaulow E, Herland OB et al (1993) Double-blind, parallel, comparative study on quality of life during treatment with amlodipine and enalapril in mild or moderate hypertensive patients: a multicenter study. J Hypertens 11:103-113
39. Omvik P, Herland OB, Thaulow E et al (1995) Evaluation and quality of life assessment of amlodipine and enalapril in patients with hypertension. J Hum Hypertens 9:17-24
40. Klocek M., Czarnecka D (2001) Impact of amlodipine and enalapril on quality of life in patients with essential hypertension. Nadciśnienie Tętnicze 1:1-8
41. Weir MR, Pristant LM, Papademetriou V et al (1996) Antihypertensive therapy and quality of life. Influence of blood pressure reduction, adverse events and prior antihypertensive therapy. Am J Hypertens 9:854-859
42. Leonetti G, Magnani B, Pessina AC et al (2002) Tolerability of long-term treatment with lercanidipine versus amlodipine and lacidipine in elderly hypertensives. Am J Hypertens 15:932-940
43. Yodfat Y, Bar-On D, Amir M et al (1996) Quality of life in normotensive compared with hypertensive men treated with isradipine or methyldopa as monotherapy or in combination with captopril: the LOMIR-MCT-IL study. J Hum Hypertens 10:117-122
44. Staessen JA, Fagard R, Thijs L et al (1997) Randomised double-blind comparison of placebo and active treatment for older patients with isolated systolic hypertension. Lancet 350:757-764
45. Fletcher AE, Bulpitt CJ, Thijs L et al (2002) Quality of life on randomized treatment for isolated systolic hypertension: results from the Syst - Eur Trial. J Hypertens 20:2069-2079
46. Bulpitt CJ, Beckett NS, Fletcher AE et al (2002) Withdrawal from treatment in the Syst-Eur Trial. J Hypertens 20:339-346
47. Croog SH, Levine S, Testa MA et al (1986) The effect of antihypertensive therapy on quality of life. N Engl J Med 314:1657-1663
48. Testa MA, Anderson RB, Nanckey JF et al (1993) Quality of life and antihypertensive therapy in men: a comparison of captopril and enalapril. N Engl J Med 328:907-913
49. Fogari R, Zoppi A, Corradi L et al (1998) Sexual function in hypertensive males treated with lisinopril and atenolol: a cross-over study. Am J Hypertens 11:1244-1247
50. Esposti LD, Di Martino M, Saragoni S et al (2004) Pharmacoeconomics of antihypertensive drug treatment: and how long patients remain on various antihypertensive therapy. J Clin Hypertens 6:76-82
51. Dahlof B, Lindholm LH, Carney S et al (1997) Main results of the losartan versus amlodipine (LOA) study on drug tolerability and psychological general well-being. LOA Study Group. J Hypertens 15:1327-1335
52. Mugellini A, Preti P, Marasi G et al (2003) Influence of valsartan and enalapril on cognitive function in elderly hypertensive patients. Am J Hypertens 16:27A
53. Fogari R, Preti P, Zoppi A et al (2004) Effect of valsartan and atenolol on sexual behavior in hypertensive postmenopausal women. Am J Hypertens 17:77-81
54. Weber MA, Barkis GL, Neutel JM et al (2003) Quality of life measured in a practice-based hypertension trial of an angiotensin receptor blocker. J Clin Hypertens 5:322-329
55. Schmidt AC, Bramlage P, Limberg R et al (2008) Quality of life in hypertension management using olmesartan in primary care. Expert Opin Pharmacother 9:1641-1653

56. Williams SA, Michelson EL, Cain VA et al (2008) An evaluation of the effects of an angiotensin receptor blocker on health-related quality of life in patients with high-normal blood pressure (prehypertension) in the Trial of Preventing Hypertension (TROPHY). J Clin Hypertens 10:436-442
57. Martell N, Luque M (2001) Doxazosin added to single-drug therapy in hypertensive patients with benign prostatic hypertrophy. J Clin Hypertens 3:218-223
58. Piha J, Kaaja R (2003) Effects of moxonidine and metoprolol in penile circulation in hypertensive men with erectile dysfunction: results of a pilot study. Intern J Impot Res 15:287-289

Quality of Life in Patients with Coronary Artery Disease

3

Marek Klocek and Kalina Kawecka-Jaszcz

3.1 Introduction

Coronary artery disease (CAD) and its consequences are significant problems in community healthcare. In Europe alone, it is estimated that CAD-associated mortality amounts to ≤ 2 million individuals per year. The frequency of CAD increases with age in both sexes, constituting an important socioeconomic problem, and is the leading cause of death and disability [1]. The main goals of treating subjects with stable angina (SA) – one of the forms of CAD – is prolonging life and improving the quality of life (QoL) [2, 3]. Most people with SA have a good prognosis. However, those at very high risk, with marked left ventricular dysfunction, congestive heart failure (CHF), and/or critical coronary artery stenosis have a significantly greater risk of death. Improved survival is relatively easy to measure by clinical means, but methods used to classify the global burden of CAD (e.g., exercise stress test) are not sufficient to measure health-related quality of life (HRQoL).

The health status of populations is most often determined using indicators such as morbidity, mortality, number of specialist consultations, number of hospitalizations, and frequency of using available healthcare. However, from the perspective of QoL, all of these methods carry restrictions. They do not offer insight into the wellbeing of the individual and the influence of disease or treatment on his/her everyday functioning. Self-rated measurement of health continues to play an ever-increasing part in evaluating the effectiveness of therapy. Additionally, interactions between the physical, emotional, and social states of the subject are important etiologic factors of disease (including CAD) [3].

To a significant extent, CAD negatively affects the functioning and everyday

M. Klocek (✉)
I Department of Cardiology and Hypertension
Jagiellonian University Medical College, Kraków, Poland
e-mail: marek.klocek@wp.pl

K. Kawecka-Jaszcz et al. (eds.), *Health-Related Quality of Life in Cardiovascular Patients*,
DOI: 10.1007/978-88-470-2769-5_3 © Springer-Verlag Italia 2013

activity of the subject. Therefore, one of the most important goals of treatment is to eliminate the symptoms associated with CAD and to improve the physical and psychosocial functioning of patients. Global evaluation of the advantages patients encounter in treatment should not overlook HRQoL. Modern trends in healthcare underline the role of individualized prevention and patient care, as well as active participation by the patient in planning therapy. Such an approach obliges the physician to consider a broad definition of QoL, ensuring incorporation of the viewpoint of the patient.

3.2 Determinants of HRQoL in Subjects with CAD

People with chronic angina experience a poorer QoL in multiple areas, including physical and emotional health [4]. Measuring HRQoL in CAD patients carries prognostic value. In a study by Boswoth et al. involving 2,800 CAD patients observed over 3.5 years, lower HRQoL measured with the Short Form Health Survey (SF-36) was related to an approximately threefold greater all-cause risk of mortality and a 3.6-fold greater risk of mortality due to CAD [5]. This relationship remained statistically important even after incorporating the advanced stages of CAD, other co-morbidities, as well as psychosocial and demographic factors. A long-term study has also confirmed observations concerning the prognostic value of rating HRQoL, whereby a lower baseline QoL after a cardiac event acts as an independent predictor of increased cardiovascular-related risk of mortality [6]. Another factor significantly associated with worsening HRQoL in CAD patients is having a low level of social support. Thus, careful monitoring of perceived QoL is an important part of patient care.

Some studies [7, 8] have found that, in individuals without CAD, the presence of risk factors for cardiovascular disease (CVD), such as hypertension, hyperlipidemia, diabetes mellitus (DM), obesity, smoking, and little or no physical activity, is associated with significantly reduced HRQoL. Additionally, HRQoL decreases proportionally to the number of risk factors or diseases present. Patients with so-called "silent" or "painless" CAD (most often females) report a good QoL [9]. This finding suggests that coronary pain plays an important part in determining HRQoL.

Cardiac syndrome X is characterized by: coronary pain with abnormal findings during stress tests (exercise or echocardiography); normal coronary arteries during angiography; significantly decreased HRQoL [10]. Changes in HRQoL in subjects with cardiac syndrome X are directly related to chest pain, whereby HRQoL declines with increasing chest pain and improves after alleviation of chest pain. One of the goals of the Women's Ischemia Syndrome Evaluation (WISE) study was to confirm significant changes in the coronary arteries in >400 women reporting chest pain using coronarography. This study found that women with chest pain but with the absence of cardiac ischemia as seen during a stress test (when undertaking echocardiography using dobutamine or single photon emission computed tomography (SPECT)) reported lower HRQoL than women without chest pain. This was independent of changes in coronary arteries confirmed by angiography (i.e., a positive diagnosis of CAD) and those without any changes (i.e., cardiac syndrome X) [10]. This finding suggested that the symptoms associated with chest pain (and not only the diagnosis of CAD based on angiography results) influence HRQoL.

In summary, for individuals with symptomatic chronic CAD, the most important determinant of HRQoL is chest pain, regardless of the degree of arterial changes. Hence, the main goals of treating SA include reducing or eliminating the symptoms of chest pain, thereby improving the prognosis. Anginal pain amplifies anxiety, leads to restrictions in physical functioning and, as a consequence, restricts the social functioning of the individual [9]. Typically, chest pain (which occurs predominantly in men) is described as a "pressure", is localized over the sternum, and often radiates to the shoulders, neck, and jaw. It can be described as "burning", "hot", "crushing", "compressing", or "squeezing". Pain may be aggravated in various ways (exercise, stress, cold). The classification system developed in the 1970s [11] by the Canadian Cardiovascular Society (CCS) has been accepted throughout the world to grade the degree of advancement of angina symptoms (Table 3.1).

Across all age groups, subjects with stable CAD who suffer angina attacks are characterized by lower HRQoL than healthy individuals [3]. The QoL of such CAD patients is 15–30% lower than that of healthy individuals of identical age, and is also lower than that of subjects with arterial hypertension or DM only [12]. Conversely, patients with CAD and concomitant diseases such as DM or chronic

Table 3.1 Functional classification of angina pectoris according to the Canadian Cardiovascular Society

Grade	Description
I	Ordinary physical activity does not cause angina, such as walking and climbing stairs. Angina with strenuous or rapid or prolonged exertion at work or recreation.
II	Slight limitation of ordinary activity. Walking or climbing stairs rapidly, walking uphill, walking or stair climbing after meals, or in cold, or in wind, or under emotional stress, or only during the few hours after awakening. Walking more than two blocks on the level and climbing more than one flight of ordinary stairs at a normal pace and in normal conditions
III	Marked limitation of ordinary physical activity. Walking one or two blocks on the level and climbing one flight of stairs in normal conditions and at normal pace produces angina.
IV	Inability to carry on any physical activity without discomfort; anginal syndrome may be present at rest.

obstructive pulmonary disease (COPD) are characterized by significantly lower HRQoL than CAD patients without concomitant health problems [13]. In general, it is accepted that the degree of advancement of CAD (in terms of progressive atherosclerotic changes) is correlated with decreased HRQoL. However, certain studies, carried out using select questionnaires commonly used to measure the HRQoL of CAD patients, did not demonstrate such a strong relationship. Thus, it seems that poor physical functioning, most often caused by angina symptoms (mainly pain and breathlessness) is not the only determinant of HRQoL in CAD.

In CAD patients, similar to those with hypertension, women reported worse general HRQoL than that observed in men [14, 15]. It is well known that women experience coronary heart disease in a different way to that experienced by men. Presentations of cardiac pain for women can include vague signs and symptoms such as extreme fatigue, discomfort in the shoulder blades, and shortness of breath. Women have a higher prevalence of functional disability and a lower prevalence of obstructive coronary heart disease (as evidenced by coronary angiography) than men [16]. The paradoxical sex difference in which women have a lower prevalence of anatomical CAD but worsening symptoms, ischemia and outcomes appears to be linked to a sex-specific pathophysiology of coronary reactivity, and includes microvascular dysfunction, which is more prevalent in women [17]. Compared with men, the reduction in the perception of HRQoL may even reach 10–20% in women [18]. Nevertheless, differences have not been found between men and women with CAD in terms of self-rated health, which has been reported by both sexes as being "average". However, more female patients than male patients feel that their everyday activities are negatively affected by CAD symptoms. Also, more female patients than male patients feel that these restrictions in everyday activity resulting from CAD have increased in the past 6 months [2]. Poor self-rated health and negative attitudes concerning illness lead to decreased HRQoL in psychological and physical dimensions. It has been reported that depression symptoms have a greater impact on the HRQoL of women with post-myocardial infarction compared with men 1 year after a cardiac incident.

Poorer self-rated health status not only has scientific value, but also has important clinical utility because it plays a part in the prognosis of women with CAD. Data from the WISE study confirmed that women with suspected myocardial ischemia who rated their health as "poor" (hazard ratio (HR): 2.1) or "fair" (HR: 2.0) experienced significantly shorter times to major CVD events compared with women who rated their health as "excellent" or "very good". In the WISE study, self-rated health predicted major CVD events independently of demographic factors, CVD risk factors, and angiography-defined disease severity [19].

Westin et al. [14] studied 400 subjects with CAD coronary after their first cardiac incident. They found that the HRQoL of women 1 month after the cardiac incident (i.e., measuring general health, anxiety, depression, self-esteem, sexual health, arrhythmia) as well as 1 year later (i.e., measuring general health, anxiety, depression) was lower than in men. Additionally, 19–45% of those studied recorded worsening HRQoL after 1 year. Careful attention should be paid to the significantly worsened HRQoL of women with CAD if undertaking the secondary prevention of SA.

Several theories have arisen concerning the sex-dependent differences in HRQoL in CAD patients and the general population. van Jaarsveld et al. [20] discovered that lower HRQoL in women suffering from CAD was explained by their greater sensitivity to changes in HRQoL resulting from increased restrictions in physical and social activity, which brought about heightened levels of stress and frustration. That finding suggested that psychological distress and role pressure were characteristic of women with CAD. A lower level of education was an additional factor negatively influencing the HRQoL of women with CAD. In the WISE study, in which the primary endpoint was evaluation of the independent contribution of socioeconomic factors on the estimation of time to cardiovascular death or myocardial infarction (MI), 819 women were enrolled and referred for clinically indicated coronary angiography. With respect to socioeconomic factors, income remained a significant predictor of cardiovascular death or MI in risk-adjusted models that controlled for angiographic coronary disease, chest-pain symptoms, and cardiac risk factors [21]. It was suggested that QoL would be more strongly associated with social support among women than in men with CAD.

Younger (i.e., aged < 55 years) male and female subjects with CAD report significantly lower self-rated health than their older counterparts. This could be because coronary disease restricts younger people from fulfilling their (usually active) professional and social roles. Advanced age is usually accompanied by less physical activity. Hence, minimal cardiac pain after percutaneous coronary intervention (PCI) or coronary artery bypass grafting (CABG) are tolerated better by older patients as opposed to more physically active younger patients. Older individuals (especially women after menopause) have less knowledge about CAD and, compared with younger individuals, take less active interest in their own health, which may influence HRQoL [22].

Atypical cardiac pain experienced by women also leads to misunderstanding of the warning signs and symptoms of MI or exacerbation of stable ischemic heart disease. Moreover, women do not recognize the threat of CAD (even if there is a significant family history) and delay seeking healthcare for signs of acute MI [16].

As in other CVDs, stark differences in HRQoL can be found between subjects with CAD and their families. Men with CAD often exaggerate the restrictions placed on them by their illness, and have a tendency to reduce their level of family and social activities. Also, family members often do not recognize the health problems of individuals with CAD. Conversely, healthy men who are partners of women with CAD tend to overstate the everyday functional restrictions of their partners. They exhibit overprotective behavior, often looking to restrict the activity of women who, as a result, feel even more "sick".

An additional factor is the psychological state and manner in which patients interpret changes to their health status. Patients who are accommodating and approach life in an optimistic manner rate their symptoms as less burdensome than do pessimistic patients, even during anginal pain [23]. An optimistic outlook ("positive affect") is associated with significantly higher HRQoL in patients subjected to different invasive procedures for treating CAD (e.g., CABG, PCI) [24]. Such an attitude is also derived from patient compliance with recommendations for therapy stated by the attending physician, as well as the patient's opinion of treatment effectiveness. On the other hand, Pelle et al. reported that CAD patients with a lack of positive affect ("anhedonia") reported poorer health status and higher levels of somatic and cognitive symptoms. Somatic and cognitive symptoms differed as a function of anhedonia over time, but health status did not [25]. In another study published recently, > 1,700 participants were observed for ≤ 10 years [26]. In this large prospective, population-based survey, positive affect (defined as the experience of pleasurable emotions such as joy, happiness, excitement, enthusiasm) was associated with a reduced risk of incident CAD independent of negative affects (depressive symptoms, hostility, anxiety). That finding underlined the protective effects of positive affect on physical health and the prognosis.

More advanced stages of chronic CAD often lead to an increased risk of MI, which is accompanied by heightened emotional stress. However, after a few months, most post-MI patients return to a stable psychological state and optimal physical functioning [27]. In ≈25–30% of such patients, a constant feeling of uneasiness concerning their health remains and/or depression develops, leading to decreased HRQoL. It has been demonstrated that the negative influence of MI on HRQoL more frequently affects younger patients (< 55 years old) and may even last ≤ 2 years after the incident.

In the Global Utilization of Streptokinase and t-PA for Occluded Coronary Arteries (GUSTO-I) Angiographic study, it was confirmed that, 2 years after MI, left ventricular ejection fraction (LVEF) correlated well with post-MI HRQoL (i.e., the lower the LVEF, the lower the HRQoL) [28]. Carrying out psychological tests and observing patients after MI allows the future course of coronary disease to be predicted. Choosing appropriate treatment (including lifestyle management) improves the prognosis and allows for a quicker return to normal activity. Schweikert et al. analyzed data from the Monitoring Trends and Determinants in Cardiovascular Disease (MONICA)/Cooperative Health Research in the Region of Augsburg (KORA) Myocardial Infarction Registry in Augsburg, Germany. That registry contains ≈2,950 patients, and they confirmed that MI survivors had a significant reduction in HRQoL (measured with the EQ-5D VAS questionnaire) compared with the general population [29]. In this study, the main predictors of lower HRQoL were older age, DM, obesity, current smoking, and experience of re-infarction. Having a heart attack at a young age (45–54 years) was particularly devastating for HRQoL: in young survivors, MI decreased HRQoL to the level of QoL observed in the general population 20 years later [29].

Symptoms of depression and anxiety are important factors influencing HRQoL in CAD. It is estimated that among patients with stable CAD, 25–45% at some point require pharmacological therapy for depression [30]. This group is even greater among post-MI patients and those with CHF. Long-term clinical studies have confirmed that individuals with CVD also suffering from depression have a 3.5-fold greater risk of death 18-months after MI than individuals without depression. Newer data further describe the influence of depression which presents after acute coronary syndrome (ACS) or during hospitalization due to ACS. In such cases, depression not only progressively decreases HRQoL, but also increases the risk of cardiovascular death ≤ 5 years after an acute cardiovascular event [31].

Hospitalization due to coronary disease is another factor associated with reduced HRQoL in certain patients. It has also been found that individuals with a reduced level of social support (material or emotional) more often present with depression and an increased level of aggression 1 month after angiographic diagnostic testing. This relationship exists irrespective of sex, age, and degree of CAD advancement.

Another study in a random group of 250 patients with CAD measuring HRQoL the Cardiac Health Profile (CHP) and the EQ-VAS questionnaires found cognitive dysfunction to be the strongest determinant of HRQoL [32]. Cognitive dysfunction (measured in terms of memory, ability to learn, and concentration) explained 43% of differences in these questionnaires and influenced HRQoL to a greater extent than a breakdown in physical and psychological wellbeing [32]. Moreover, the degree of cognitive dysfunction was independent of the CCS class presented by the patients.

Data obtained from the Translational Research Investigating Underlying Disparities in Recovery from Acute Myocardial Infarction: Patients' Health Status (TRIUMPII) Registry in the USA have shown that cognitive impairment without dementia (CIND) occurs in > 50% of older adult survivors of acute MI [33]. Moreover, in older CAD patients (mean age, 73 years), CIND was associated with less invasive care, less referral and participation in cardiac rehabilitation, and worse risk-adjusted 1-year survival.

3.3 Methods Used to Measure QoL in Subjects with CAD

Assessing the HRQoL of CAD patients has been measured using general and specific questionnaires. HRQoL measures can be classified as "generic" (covering health in general) or "disease-specific", and typically address various dimensions of health, including physical functioning, social and emotional functioning, perceived health status, life satisfaction, and interpersonal relationships. The most often used generic questionnaires include the Short Form 36-item Survey (SF-36), Sickness Impact Profile (SIP), Quality of Well Being Scale (QWB), EuroQoL-5D (EQ-5D), Nottingham Health Profile (NHP) and Quality of Life Index-Cardiac Version III (QLI). The most often used specific questionnaires include the Seattle Angina Questionnaire (SAQ), Health Complaints Scale in Coronary Artery Disease (HCS-CAD), MacNew Heart Disease Health-Related Quality of Life Questionnaire (MacNew), Quality of Life After Myocardial Infarction (QLMI), Angina Pectoris Quality of Life Questionnaire (SAQLQ), Cardiac Health Profile (CHP), Angina-related Limitations at Work Questionnaire, Cardiovascular Limitations and Symptoms Profile (CLASP), and Myocardial Infarction Dimensional Assessment Scale (MIDAS) (see Appendix).

Dougherty et al. [34] compared the SAQ, SF-36, and QLMI in 107 patients with SA: 97 (90.6%) received a calcium antagonist, 86 (80.4%) nitrates, and 56 (52.3%) beta-blockers. This study found that the severity of SA (measured using the CCS scale) could be correlated to all categories of the SAQ, two categories of the SF-36, and none of the QLMI scales. All these instruments gave similar results if readministered to the same patients 2 weeks later. The SAQ is specially designed for CAD patients and measures the physical state, symptom severity, and subjective HRQoL.

Visser et al. [35] also used questionnaires to study the HRQoL of CAD patients: SIP, NHP, and QWB. These results were correlated with CAD stage based on the New York Health Association (NYHA) scale. Included in this study were 59 patients presenting with SA. When comparing these questionnaires against increasing NYHA stages, 4 out of 6 symptom groups were seen to increase in severity in the NHP, 6 out of 11 groups increased in severity in the SIP, and only 2 out of 4 groups increased in severity in the QWB questionnaire. The QWB questionnaire was also the most difficult to use, giving the least reliable results due to high variability across 3 individuals to whom the questionnaire was administered. This questionnaire was also least sensitive to changes in the degree of angina symptoms. NHP and SIP questionnaires gave highly correlated results ($r = 0.82$, $p < 0.001$) in similar categories (e.g., emotional status or sleep quality). The coefficients of variation were also lower in the NHP and SIP questionnaires. The authors concluded that these two questionnaires were valuable tools for measuring the effects of therapy on CAD patients.

Not all generic questionnaires are sufficiently sensitive to be used to detect changes in the health status of CAD patients. Thus, with the aim of measuring HRQoL in this group of patients, it is necessary to use a combination of generic and specific questionnaires [36]. The vast number of questionnaires used to measure HRQoL in CAD patients does not simplify study design, nor does it allow for easy comparison of data. Hence, in 2005, the European Society of Cardiology began the Euro Cardio-QoL Project. This was implemented in 15 European countries with the aim of developing a reliable questionnaire ("HeartQoL") to measure HRQoL in CAD patients [37]. The project is ongoing.

3.4 Influence of Treatment on the HRQoL of Subjects with CAD

Treatment of SA is multidirectional and usually involves correction of several risk factors (i.e., lifestyle modification), pharmacological management, invasive procedures (e.g., coronary revascularization), prevention of sudden cardiac death, and treating concomitant diseases. The main goals of SA treatment include reducing or eliminating chest-pain symptoms and improving the prognosis through secondary prevention. In recent years, it has also been found that aspirin and hypolipidemic drugs markedly decrease the risk of MI, hospitalization, and mortality in this group of patients.

3.5 Effects of Catheters or Surgery

PCI is considered to be the first-line treatment for symptomatic CAD in younger and older patients, and positively influences HRQoL. Reinfret et al. [38] found that, compared with balloon angioplasty, PCI with stent implantation in acute MI led to considerable improvement in HRQoL immediately after the procedure as well as in long-term observation. However, in the Optimum Percutaneous Transluminal Coronary Angioplasty Compared with Routine Stent Strategy (OPUS-1) study, no differences were noted in HRQoL (measured using the SAQ questionnaire) in patients treated with balloon angioplasty or stent implantation [39]. Nevertheless, the HRQoL of both groups increased significantly after intervention. The results of the Randomized Intervention Trial of Unstable Angina (RITA-3) study [40] described the benefits of carrying out revascularization in patients with unstable angina or in MI patients without ST elevation. This study reported that such a procedure improved HRQoL (measured using EQ-5D, SF-36, and SAQ) more so than undertaking an invasive intervention (e.g., PCI) after having CAD symptoms for a period of time or using pharmacological treatment alone. These results mimic those of earlier studies examining improvement in HRQoL after the treatment of symptomatic CAD with invasive interventions undertaken at earlier stages.

Restenosis is a significant factor that restricts patient functioning after PCI [41]. A study using two questionnaires to measure QoL in CAD patients – the PGWB Index as a general measure and the HCS in CHD as a disease-specific measure

– found significantly lower HRQoL 6 months after restenosis in those who had previously undergone dilation of chronically occluded coronary arteries. In this group, successful revascularization with stent implantation led to improved wellbeing, decreased emotional discomfort, and increased vitality. Moreover, a reduced frequency of health-related complaints and subjective coronary symptoms was reported in the group of successfully treated patients (i.e., without restenosis of the coronary vessel) [42].

From the viewpoint of HRQoL, there are advantages and disadvantages to the different options of CAD treatment. CABG decreases or eliminates the symptoms of chest pain, improves patient functioning, and decreases the need for pharmacotherapy. Improvement in function, especially physical [43], is most often long-term and supports improvement in HRQoL [44], which may even be greater after PCI. However, after CABG, 5–15% of patients report worse HRQoL than before the procedure. This may result from postoperative pain, sleep disturbance, memory problems, and disrupted family relationships [45].

The HRQoL of patients after PCI may quickly deteriorate because of recurring angina symptoms resulting from restenosis. Recurring symptoms of chest pain or the anxiety associated with the potential of recurring coronary pain lead to decreased HRQoL in patients after PCI.

3.6 Effects of Pharmacological Treatment

Beta-blockers used in the treatment of CAD help reduce chest-pain symptoms and simultaneously yield an antihypertensive and antiarrhythmic effect. A new generation of beta-blockers may positively influence the HRQoL of patients due to lower prevalence of side effects such as bradyarrhythmia, bronchospasm, impotence, depressed mood, and nightmares.

Long-acting nitrates contribute minimally to improving the HRQoL of CAD patients [46]. Their positive influence may be reduced if, during treatment, the patient presents with dizziness, headaches, or hypotension. It has also been suggested that trimetazidine [47] improves HRQoL in selected groups of patients.

In recent years, it has also been found that angiotensin-converting enzyme inhibitors play a significant part in CAD treatment. Using perindopril in patients at moderate risk and ramipril in patients at high risk of cardiovascular events reduces the prevalence of death, MI and stroke. However, there is a lack of data concerning the influence of these drugs on the HRQoL of subjects with symptomatic CAD.

With respect to the prognosis, decreasing symptoms of chest pain and improving HRQoL, invasive revascularization methods (PCI (with and without stenting), CABG) are advantageous compared with pharmacological treatment of symptomatic

CAD [48]. However, not all CAD patients are suitable candidates for revascularization. Those who are treated with pharmacotherapy alone have especially low HRQoL and require careful medical attention [49].

As part of cardiologic rehabilitation, physical training over a few months improves HRQoL in diverse groups of CAD patients (especially in those who have suffered MI). It has been found that systematic physical training helps reduce weight in obese patients, improves physical endurance, decreases cholesterol levels, and reduces anxiety and depression. These factors relate to a sizable percentage of post-MI patients and those with SA, including those who have undergone CABG [50].

References

1. Leal J, Luengo-Fernandez R, Gray A et al (2006) Economic burden of cardiovascular diseases in the enlarged European Union. Eur Heart J 27:1610-1619
2. Swenson JR, Clinch J (2000) Assessment of quality of life in patients with cardiac disease: the role of psychosomatic medicine. J Psychosom Res 48:405-415
3. Brink E, Grankvist G, Karlson BW et al (2005) Health-related quality of life in women and men one year after acute myocardial infarction. Qual Life Res 14:749-757
4. Kimble LP, Dunbar SB, Weintraub WS et al (2011) Symptom clusters and health-related quality of life in people with chronic stable angina. J Adv Nurs 67:1000-1011
5. Bosworth HB, Siegler IC, Brummet BH et al (1999) The association between self-rated health and mortality in a well-characterized sample of coronary artery disease patients. Med Care 37:1226-1236
6. Westin L, Nilstun T, Carlsson R et al (2005) Patients with ischemic heart disease: quality of life predicts long-term mortality. Scand Cardiovasc J 39:50-54
7. Lalonde L, Clarke AE, Joseph L et al (2001) Health-related quality of life in coronary heart disease prevention and treatment. J Clin Epidemiol 54:1011-1018
8. Lalonde L, O'Connor A, Joseph L et al (2004) Health-related quality of life in cardiac patients with dyslipidemia and hypertension. Qual Life Res 13:793-804
9. Olson MB, Kelsey SF, Matthews K et al (2003) Symptoms, myocardial ischaemia and quality of life in women: Results from the NHLBI-sponsored WISE Study. Eur Heart J 24:1506-1514
10. Asbury EA, Collins P (2005) Psychosocial factors associated with noncardiac chest pain and cardiac syndrome X. Herz 30:55-60
11. Campeau L (2002) The Canadian Cardiovascular Society grading of angina pectoris revisited 30 years later. Can J Cardiol 18:371-379
12. Alonso J, Ferrer M, Gandek B et al (2004) Health-related quality of life associated with chronic conditions in eight countries: Results from the International Quality of Life Assessment (IQOLA) Project. Qual Life Res 13:283-298
13. Pischke CR, Weidner G, Elliott-Eller M et al (2006) Comparison of coronary risk factors and quality of life in coronary artery disease patients with versus without diabetes mellitus. Am J Cardiol 97:1267-1273
14. Westin L, Carlsson R, Erhardt L et al (1999) Differences in quality of life in men and women with ischemic heart disease. A prospective controlled study. Scand Cardiovasc J 33:160-165
15. Dueñas M, Ramirez C, Arana R et al (2011) Gender differences and determinants of health related quality of life in coronary patients: a follow-up study. BMC Cardiovasc Disord 11:24
16. O'Keefe-McCarthy S (2008) Women's experiences of cardiac pain: a review of the literature. Can J Cardiovasc Nurs 18:18-25

17. Merz CN, Shaw LJ (2011) Stable angina in women: lessons from the National Heart, Lung and Blood Institute-sponsored Women's Ischemia Syndrome Evaluation. J Cardiovasc Med 12:85-87
18. Norris CM, Ghali WA, Galbraith PD et al (2004) Women with coronary artery disease report worse health-related quality of life outcomes compared to men. Health & Quality of Life Outcomes 2:21
19. Rutledge T, Linke SE, Johnson BD et al (2010) Self-rated versus objective health indicators as predictors of major cardiovascular events: the NHLBI-sponsored Women's Ischemia Syndrome Evaluation. Psychosom Med 72:549-555
20. Van Jaarsveld CHM, Sanderman R, Ranchor AV et al (2002) Gender-specific changes in quality of life following cardiovascular disease. A prospective study. J Clin Epidemiol 55:1005-1112
21. Shaw LJ, Merz CN, Bittner V et al (2008) Importance of socioeconomic status as a predictor of cardiovascular outcome and costs of care in women with suspected myocardial ischemia. Results from the National Institutes of Health, National Heart, Lung and Blood Institute-sponsored Women's Ischemia Syndrome Evaluation (WISE). J Womens Health 17:1081-1092
22. French DP, Lewin RJP, Watson N et al (2005) Do illness perceptions predict attendance at cardiac rehabilitation and quality of life following myocardial infarction? J Psychosom Res 59:315-322
23. Steele A, Wade TD (2004) The contribution of optimism and quality of life to depression in an acute coronary syndrome population. Eur J Cardiovasc Nurs 3:231-237
24. Versteeg H, Pedersen SS, Erdman RAM et al (2009) Negative and positive affect are independently associated with patient-reported health status following percutaneous coronary intervention. Qual Life Res 18:953-960
25. Pelle AJ, Pedersen SS, Erdman RAM et al (2011) Anhedonia is associated with poor health status and more somatic and cognitive symptoms in patients with coronary artery disease. Qual Life Res 20:643-651
26. Davidson KW, Mostofsky E, Whang W (2010) Don't worry, be happy: positive affect and reduced 10-year incident coronary heart disease: The Canadian Nova Scotia Health Survey. Eur Heart J 31:1065-1070
27. Beck CA, Joseph L, Belisle P, Pilote L (2001) Predictors of quality of life 6 months and 1 year after myocardial infarction. Am Heart J 142:271-279
28. Coyne KS, Lundergan CF, Boyle D et al (2000) Relationship of infarct artery patency and left ventricular ejection fraction to health-related quality of life after myocardial infarction. The GUSTO-I angiographic study experience. Circulation 102:1245-1251
29. Schweikert B, Hunger M, Meisinger Ch et al (2009) Quality of life several years after myocardial infarction: comparing MONICA/KORA registry to the general population. Eur Heart J 30:436-443
30. Dobbels F, De Guest S, Vanhees L et al (2002) Depression and the heart: a systematic overview of definition, measurement, consequences and treatment of depression in cardiovascular disease. Eur J Cardiovasc Nurs 1:45-55
31. Grace SL, Abbey SE, Kapral MK et al (2005) Effect of depression on five-year mortality after an acute coronary syndrome. Am J Cardiol 96:1179-1185
32. Kiessling A, Henriksson P (2004) Perceived cognitive function is a major determinant of health-related quality of life in a non-selected population of patients with coronary artery disease – a principal components analysis. Qual Life Res 13:1621-1631
33. Gharacholou SM, Reid KJ, Arnold SV et al (2011) Cognitive impairment and outcomes in older adult survivors of acute myocardial infarction: Findings from the Translational Research investigating Underlying disparities in acute Myocardial Infarction Patients' Health Status registry. Am Heart J 162:860-869
34. Dougherty CM, Dewhurst T, Nichol WP et al (1998) Comparison of three quality of life instruments in stable angina pectoris: the Seattle Angina Questionnarie (SAQ), the Short Form Health Survey (SF-36) and the Quality of Life Index-Cardiac Version III (QLI). J Clin Epidemiol 51:569-575

35. Visser MC, Fletcher AE, Parr G et al (1994) A comparison of three quality of life instruments in subjects with angina pectoris: the Sickness Impact Profile, the Nottingham Health Profile and the Quality of Well Being Scale. J Clin Epidemiol 47:157-163
36. Thompson DR, Roebuck A (2001) The measurement of health-related quality of life in patients with coronary heart disease. J Cardiovasc Nurs 16:28-33
37. Oldridge N, Saner H, McGee HM (2005) The Euro Cardio-QoL Project. An international study to develop a core heart disease health-related quality of life questionnaire, the HeartQoL. Eur J Cardiovasc Prev Rehab 12:87-94
38. Rinfret S, Grines CL, Cosgove S et al (2001) Quality of life after balloon angioplasty or stenting for acute myocardial infarction: one-year results from the Stent-PAMI trial. J Am Coll Cardiol 38:1614-1621
39. Weaver WD, Reisman MA, Griffin JJ et al (2000) Optimum percutaneous transluminal coronary angioplasty compared with routine stent strategy trial (OPUS-1): a randomised trial. Lancet 355:2199-2203
40. Kim J, Henderson RA, Pocock SJ et al (2005) Health-related quality of life after interventional or conservative strategy in patients with unstable angina or non-ST segment elevation myocardial infarction. One-year results of the third randomized intervention trial of unstable angina (RITA-3). J Am Coll Cardiol 45:221-228
41. Odell A, Grip L, Hallberg LR (2006) Restenosis after percutaneous coronary intervention (PCI): experiences from the patients' perspective. Eur J Cardiovasc Nurs 5:150-157
42. Bryniarski L (2005) Optimization of revascularization of chronic total coronary occlusions. Jagiellonian University Press, Kraków
43. Szygula-Jurkiewicz B, Zembala M, Wilczek K (2005) Health related quality of life after percutaneous coronary intervention versus coronary artery bypass graft surgery in patients with acute coronary syndromes without ST-segment elevation. 12-month follow up. Eur J Cardio-Thor Surg 27:882-886
44. Brorsson B, Bernstein SJ, Brook RH et al (2001) Quality of life of chronic stable angina patients 4 years after coronary angioplasty or coronary artery bypass surgery. J Inter Med 249:47-57
45. Hunt JO, Hendrata MV, Myles PS (2000) Quality of life 12 months after coronary artery bypass graft surgery. Heart Lung 29:401-411
46. Spertus JA, Dewhurst T, Dougherty CM et al (2001) Testing the effectiveness of converting patients to long-acting antianginal medications: The Quality of Life in Angina Research Trial (QUART). Am Heart J 141:550-558
47. Vitale C, Wajngaten M, Sposato B et al (2004) Trimetazidine improves left ventricular function and quality of life in elderly patients with coronary artery disease. Eur Heart J 25:1814-1821
48. Lukkarinen H, Hentinen M (2006) Treatments of coronary artery disease improve quality of life in the long term. Nurs Res 55:26-33
49. Lenzen M, Scholte op Reimer W, Norekval TM et al (2006) Pharmacological treatment and perceived health status during 1-year follow-up in patients diagnosed with coronary artery disease, but ineligible for revascularization. Results from the Euro Heart Survey on Coronary Revascularization. Eur J Cardiovasc Nurs 5:115-121
50. Hung C, Daub B, Black B et al (2004) Exercise training improves overall physical fitness and quality of life in older women with coronary artery disease. Chest 126:1026-1031

Quality of Life in Patients After Coronary Interventional Treatment

4

Leszek Bryniarski and Marek Klocek

4.1 Introduction

A long-term goal of treating coronary artery disease (CAD) is to decrease mortality by reducing the prevalence of myocardial infarction (MI) and sudden cardiac death. An immediate goal of treatment is to minimize chest pain (coronary pain, angina), increase physical tolerance, and to positively influence the quality of life (QoL) of patients by alleviating symptoms [1].

CAD is one of the most often encountered diseases in the world. From 1950 to 1990, an increase in the incidence of new-onset CAD was documented in many countries, and a rise in mortality observed. However, these negative trends have been reversed during the last two decades in many countries. For instance, in young adults, mortality due to CAD and cerebrovascular disease has steadily declined in Europe [2]. Also, in the USA and Canada, mortality due to CAD has declined by ≈60% in both sexes [3]. Conversely, there is a tendency for increased morbidity due to CAD in aging populations.

Coronary pain is a main determinant of health-related quality of life (HRQoL) in CAD patients. The presence and severity of angina negatively influences various dimensions of health status and everyday functioning. Poor physical health has been shown to be an important predictor for a poor prognosis in patients with CAD treated with percutaneous coronary interventions [4]. Differences in the impairment of HRQoL associated with CAD have been noted across different age, racial and ethnic groups [5]. The side effects of long-term pharmacotherapy (especially in those using many drugs every day) may also adversely affect HRQoL, and result in noncompliance during therapy. Percutaneous coronary intervention (PCI) and coronary

L. Bryniarski (✉)
I Department of Cardiology and Hypertension
Jagiellonian University Medical College, Kraków, Poland
e-mail: l_bryniarski@poczta.fm

K. Kawecka-Jaszcz et al. (eds.), *Health-Related Quality of Life in Cardiovascular Patients*,
DOI: 10.1007/978-88-470-2769-5_4

artery bypass grafting (CABG) decrease the frequency of chest pain, improve health, and prolong the life of CAD patients. Though costly (with patients undergoing PCI sometimes needing to repeat the procedure due to restenosis), these interventions are advantageous because of their influence on HRQoL.

Myocardial revascularization has been an established mainstay for the treatment of CAD for several years. CABG has been used in since the 1960s, and is arguably the most intensively studied surgical procedure ever undertaken. PCI has been used since the 1980s. It has been subjected to more randomized clinical trials than any other interventional procedure [6].

CABG and PCI have witnessed significant technological advances, in particular the use of drug-eluting stents (DES) in PCI and of arterial grafts in CABG. However, their role in the treatment of subjects presenting with stable CAD is being challenged by advances in medical treatment (referred to as "optimal medical therapy"), which includes intensive lifestyle management and pharmacological management. Furthermore, differences between the two revascularization strategies should be recognized. In CABG, bypass grafts are placed to the coronary vessel beyond the "culprit" lesion(s), thereby providing extra sources of nutrient blood flow to the myocardium and offering protection against the consequences of further proximal obstructive disease. In contrast, PCI with coronary stents aims to restore the normal conductance of the native coronary vasculature without offering protection against new disease proximal to the stent [6].

4.2 PCI in Stable Angina

Stable angina pectoris is a main syndrome of chronic CAD. Usually, PCI is undertaken in patients with refractory or progressing angina attacks. However, PCI does not significantly decrease mortality in stable angina [7]. Despite the many PCI procedures undertaken worldwide, few studies have examined the long-term effects on the HRQoL of patients after this procedure, as seen in everyday clinical practice [8]. However, in general, we can conclude that PCIs improve HRQoL in subjects with stable angina pectoris, as discussed below.

The HRQoL of patients subject to revascularization (percutaneous and surgical) is significantly higher than in patients treated conservatively [8]. In a 10-year study, Westin et al. found that self-rated HRQoL is of prognostic value for estimating the risk of death after a cardiac event (MI, CABG, angioplasty) [9]. Surprisingly, the increase in HRQoL did not produce an increase in survival [7].

Compared with pharmacotherapy, revascularization in subjects with stable angina decreases chest pain to a greater extent and objectively decreases myocardial ischemia [7]. A study examining the options of invasive CAD treatment found that patients were familiar with this form of therapy. Hence, carrying out the procedure has a very large placebo effect [1]. Physicians often concentrate on the "hard" endpoints (e.g., mortality) and have a tendency to not appreciate the complaints of patients. However, from the patients' perspective, restrictions in everyday functioning are of the greatest significance, either at home or during professional activities.

The Angioplasty Compared to Medicine (ACME) study found significant improvement in the HRQoL of men treated by PCI for single-vessel coronary disease, but did not find as significant a improvement in patients with double-vessel disease [10]. Spertus et al. examined the relationship between the baseline characteristics of 1,518 post-MI patients and their HRQoL 1 year after PCI [11]. Improvement in HRQoL was proportional to the severity of angina before the procedure. Using the Seattle Angina Questionnaire (SAQ), significant improvement was noted in those with, as compared with those without, angina. Scores increased by 21.4 ± 2.1 points in patients with symptomatic angina once per month, by 30.7 ± 2.2 points in those presenting with symptoms once per week, and by 34.6 ± 2.6 points in those with everyday angina pain. Improvement in patient HRQoL was also dependent upon age. The ACME study once again confirmed the fundamental role of coronary pain as a restrictive factor in the HRQoL of CAD patients. Among patients without angina, 36% noted significant improvement in HRQoL, whereas improvement was noted in 85% of patients with angina [11]. PCI also leads to improvement in the HRQoL of asymptomatic CAD patients.

The main results of the Clinical Outcomes Utilizing Revascularization and Aggressive Drug Evaluation (COURAGE) Trial were published in 2007 [12]. In this trial, 2,287 patients with stable angina pectoris were randomly assigned to PCI with optimal medical therapy or to optimal medical therapy alone. The design and results of the trial aroused controversy. The design of the COURAGE Trial had two main problems: (i) it did not meet pre-specified assumptions about statistical power despite protocol changes made after the trial was underway that placed PCI at a disadvantage; and (ii) only a small percentage of screened patients were included, revascularization was incomplete, and 32% of the medical therapy group needed revascularization. In 2008, the results of QoL components in the COURAGE Trial were published [13]. Angina-specific health status (with the use of the SAQ) and overall physical and mental function (with use of the 36-item Short Form Health Survey (SF-36)) were assessed. At 3 months, 53% of patients in the PCI group and 42% in the medical-therapy group remained angina-free. By 3 months, SAQ scores had increased in the PCI group as compared with the optimal medical therapy group for: physical limitations ($p = 0.004$); angina stability ($p = 0.002$); angina frequency ($p < 0.001$); treatment satisfaction ($p < 0.001$); and QoL ($p < 0.001$). In general, patients had an incremental benefit from PCI for 6 months to 24 months. Patients with more severe angina had a greater benefit from PCI. Similar benefits from PCI were seen in some (but not all) domains of the SF-36. However, by 36 months, there was no significant difference in health status between the treatment groups. The authors concluded that patients with stable CAD, both those treated with PCI and those treated with optimal medical therapy alone, had marked improvements in health status during follow-up. The PCI group had small (but significant) incremental benefits in the early post-intervention period that disappeared by 36 months after intervention. However, the COURAGE Trial was not a "head-to-head" study of PCI versus optimal medical therapy, but instead a strategy comparison of upfront PCI with optimal medical therapy versus upfront optimal medical therapy alone. Most of the patients who received optimal medical therapy alone had improved symptoms within 3 months, but 21% crossed over and received PCI. Thus, the COURAGE Trial revealed that the treatment of patients with stable angina should be started with optimal medical therapy but, if this is ineffective, use PCI. The COURAGE Trial also showed the value of integrating measures of health status (such as the SAQ) in routine clinical practice. In particular, the PCI-first strategy provided the largest benefit for those with a SAQ score < 50 points (corresponding to those having angina several times a week). In contrast, those with higher scores in the SAQ (less frequent or no angina) had less benefit or no benefit from upfront PCI. These findings showed that measures of health status may be useful to select a treatment option and to monitor its effectiveness [14].

Several studies have looked at the influence of PCI on HRQoL, but only a few have examined the relationship between the baseline characteristics of patients and improvement in HRQoL after PCI [15, 16]. However, most data come from cross-sectional studies which incorporate a supplementary measure of symptoms presented by the patient and the influence of these symptoms on HRQoL. These were not prospective studies conducted with the aim of measuring HRQoL. Permanyer-Miralda et al. found that, in a group of 106 patients, residual angina after PCI was the most important determinant of decreased HRQoL 3 years after angioplasty [17]. Similarly, Pocock et al. confirmed the significant relationship between the influence of angina, shortness of breath, and limited exercise tolerance on HRQoL for 1 year after the procedure [18]. None of these studies concentrated on the determinants of patient HRQoL before the procedure. Hence, Nash et al. examined the baseline predictors of QoL in 1,182 patients before angioplasty [19]. They found that poor HRQoL at baseline (low physical component (PCS) and low mental component (MCS) scores on SF-36) acted as an independent determinant of improvement from angioplasty 6 months after the procedure.

Similar results were obtained in the study by de Quadros et al. [20]. Patients with stable angina (n = 110) were assessed by the SAQ before PCI and followed up for 1 year. Authors revealed that there was an improvement in all SAQ scales after 1 year in most patients treated with PCI in the "real-world practice" (68% of patients were free of angina 1 year after PCI). In multivariate analyses, QoL before the procedure was the main positive predictor of improvement in QoL. This study confirmed the positive impact of PCI on symptom relief in chronic stable angina in everyday clinical practice.

The number of elderly patients is increasing worldwide and require special attention. The Trial of Invasive Versus Medical Therapy in Elderly Patients (TIME) compared two strategies for treating symptomatic, stable angina in patients aged ≥ 75 years. Results confirmed that an invasive diagnostic approach (coronography) and, depending on the result, PCI or CABG, significantly improved HRQoL 6 months after the procedure [21]. This improvement was similar for men and women with CAD despite the lower overall scores for women [22]. However, after 1 year, no significant differences in mortality, MI, or symptom improvement were noted between conservative and invasive strategies. This was primarily because, at this time, 43% of patients who initially qualified for pharmacological treatment underwent revascularization because of recurring angina. The TIME study, which looked at individuals aged ≥ 75 years, attained similar results to those in the Randomised Intervention Treatment of Angina (RITA-2) study [23], which examined younger CAD patients with a mean age of 58 years. In both age groups, early improvement in angina symptoms and HRQoL after invasive treatment for CAD (i.e., PCI or CABG) disappeared with time, after 1 year. Conversely, younger and older CAD patients treated conservatively were found to: have a greater incidence of non-fatal cardiovascular episodes and hospitalizations; use more anti-anginal drugs; require revascularization more often [24]. Hence, their HRQoL was poor.

In another study, using SF-36 and SAQ , Seto et al. did not find differences based on age in HRQoL after PCI [25]. At observation times of 6 months and 12 months, they authors found similar levels of HRQoL in 295 patients aged ≥ 70 years as in 1,150 patients aged < 70 years.

Li et al. observed 624 elderly subjects with acute coronary syndromes (ACS) admitted to hospital [26]. HRQoL was assessed at baseline and after 6 months by SF-36. The authors found that HRQoL at baseline decreased with advancing age. However, even though older patients were less likely to undergo angioplasty (56% of patients aged 60–79 years versus 21% of patients aged > 80 years), subjects from the older group who underwent PCI experienced the most improvement in physical health as compared with younger ones. The investigators suggested that age should not be an argument against coronary revascularization with PCI due to the potential benefits in HRQoL.

However, one may suppose that, with a decreased incidence of restenosis after the introduction of DES compared with that encountered with bare metal stents (BMS), and the consequent decrease in recurring anginal symptoms, such stents should lead to improvement in HRQoL [36, 37]. Recently published data from the Rapamycin-Eluting Stent Evaluated at Rotterdam Cardiology Hospital (RESEARCH) Registry can partially address this issue [27]. More than 800 consecutive patients (mean age, 62 years) treated with PCI with implantations of sirolimus-eluting stents (SES) or BMS were involved. At inclusion, ≈50% of participants suffered from stable angina. Patients were not randomized to stent type. HRQoL was measured with SF-36, and 59% of patients had good health status at 1 month and 12 months after PCI. Poor health status at baseline was predictive of higher mortality at 6-year follow-up, and this effect was independent of demographic and clinical characteristics. The results of this study showed that patient-reported health status should be adopted in standard clinical practice for identification of high-risk CAD patients, who will be (or already have been) treated with DES.

Pedersen et al. also assessed the impact of patient-rated health status on the prognosis in subjects treated with PCI with paclitaxel-eluting stents (PES) [28]. Eight-hundred and seventy CAD patients completed the EuroQoL-5D (EQ-5D) questionnaire just after PCI. Two dimensions of the questionnaire, "mobility" and "self-care" as well as self-reported health status as measured with the EQ visual analog scale (EQ VAS) scale were independent predictors of death or MI at 1-year follow-up (more than twofold risk).

4.3 PCI and CABG in Multivessel CAD

Large-scale clinical studies comparing CABG and PCI with pharmacological treatment reported that any reduction in mortality is proportional to the degree of disease progression [7]. Only in the case of left main stenosis or triple-vessel CAD (especially with left ventricular contractile dysfunction) does CABG extend patient survival. Recently published data indicate that implantation of DES can provide similar long-term survival in multivessel CAD [29].

Earlier studies showed the superiority of CABG over PCI in terms of extending short- and long-term survival as well as improving HRQoL. Hlatky et al. [30] compared the results of the Bypass Angioplasty Revascularization Investigation (BARI) study with the Study of Economics and Quality of Life (SEQOL). The BARI study took place before the era of stents (i.e., only balloon angioplasty was done) and involved 934 patients with multivessel CAD randomized to CABG or PCI who simultaneously took part in the SEQOL. The authors found that, compared with PCI, HRQoL improved most significantly in the first 3 years after CABG, and that this difference disappeared gradually after 10–12 years [30]. They also confirmed the negative influence of angina on HRQoL.

The Stent or Surgery (SoS) study examined 488 patients with multivessel CAD treated using PCI with stenting and 500 patients treated with CABG. This study found improvement in both groups with regard to health status (i.e., improved physical activity, decreased prevalence of recurrent angina) and HRQoL measured 6 months and 12 months after the intervention using the SAQ. However, improvement in HRQoL and anginal symptoms was significantly greater in patients who underwent CABG [31]. The greatest difference between PCI and CABG was observed after 6 months.

In the Medicine, Angioplasty, or Surgery Study (MASS-II), 542 patients were randomly assigned to CABG (175 subjects), PCI (180 subjects) or to standard pharmacological therapy (187 subjects) and HRQoL assessed by SF-36. All three therapeutic strategies presented significant improvements in all dimensions of the SF-36 during follow-up. However, in the CABG group, greater improvement in physical and social functioning as well as in vitality and general health was observed when compared with patients treated by pharmacological means or PCI. Also, men had higher HRQoL at the beginning of the trial when compared with women, with progressive improvement after 6 months and 12 months [32].

Attention has been drawn to differences in morbidity due to CAD between men and women. Sex seems to play a part in the effects of revascularization. The Arterial Revascularization Therapy Study (ARTS) confirmed the positive influence of CABG on HRQoL, more so than using PCI with stenting, whereas no differences were observed between men and women [33]. Zhang et al. analyzed the results of the SoS study in a group of 206 women and 782 men diagnosed with multivessel CAD randomly assigned to CABG or PCI with stenting. After 1 year, men who underwent CABG were found to have better tolerance for physical activity, decreased frequency of angina, and higher general HRQoL than men who underwent PCI. The superiority of CABG over PCI could not be confirmed in women, in whom improvement after both forms of revascularization was identical [34]. As mentioned above, the SoS study measured HRQoL at baseline as well as 6 months and 12 months after the intervention. It was measured using the SAQ, with three subscales measuring physical restrictions, frequency of angina, and HRQoL. At baseline, women in this study were older, sicker, and had lower SAQ scores than men (i.e., worse HRQoL). After 6 months, the results of SAQ testing significantly improved for men and women, especially in CABG patients. For men, with respect to physical restrictions, grafting led to greater improvement than PCI by 54.7%, by 31.3% in terms of reducing the frequency of angina, and by 18.3% for improvement in general QoL. For women, these differences were 11.6%, 43.2%, and 39.3%, respectively. One year after the procedure, men subject to CABG were found to have a greater improvement in health status than after PCI: physical restrictions improved by 50.6%, the prevalence of angina improved by 19.7%, and general HRQoL improved by 15.3%. However, differences in scores at 1 year between the two procedures decreased significantly in women to 1.6%, 11.1%, and 0.6%, respectively [33]. This was due to significant later improvement after PCI. This means that, after 1 year follow-up, CABG was advantageous for improving HRQoL only in men. In women, both procedures seemed to yield a similar benefit after 1 year. However, the limitations of this study are often raised. Firstly, there were many fewer women than men in the study. Secondly, patients' knowledge of the chosen treatment option may have influenced their answers on the SAQ. Finally, the randomization procedure meant that the sample population may not have been representative of patients with multivessel CAD.

The results of the Arterial Revascularization Therapies Study (ARTS II) compared the safety and effectiveness of patients with multivessel CAD using PCI with SES stents against the results of the ARTS I study [35]. The multicenter ARTS II involved 607 patients, with an average of 3.7 stents implanted per patient. One-year survival was very high: 99.05%. In addition, 1-year survival without stroke or MI reached 96.9%, and 1-year survival without without revascularization reached 91.5%. As the primary endpoint, 1-year survival without major adverse cardiovascular or cerebral events (MACE) reached 89.5%. The results of ARTS II were then compared with those of ARTS I. With respect to both segments of ARTS I (i.e., ARTS I – CABG and ARTS I – PCI), the reduction in relative risk (RR) for the endpoints of the study was: survival without revascularization: RR 2.03 (95% confidence interval (CI): 1.23–3.34) for CABG and 0.44 (95% CI: 0.31–0.61) for PCI; survival without MACE: RR 0.89 (95% CI: 0.65–1.23) and 0.39 (95% CI: 0.30–0.51), respectively. The results of ARTS II suggest that treating multivessel CAD with PCI using SES is safe and effective. The 3-year follow-up of this study suggested that PCI using SES seems to be safer and more efficacious than PCI using BMS irrespective of the presence of diabetes mellitus (DM) [36]. Comparison with the results of ARTS I revealed that surgical treatment continued to be related to a decreased need for revascularization. The general number of MACE in the ARTS II – PCI group was similar to that of the CABG group and significantly lower than that in the ARTS I – BMS group.

In 2010, the investigators of ARTS II published results regarding HRQoL and anginal status in patients with multivessel disease treated with PCI with SES. HRQoL outcomes were compared with the findings of ARTS I. HRQoL was evaluated at baseline and at 1, 6, 12 and 36 months after revascularization using SF-36. The analyzed groups were treated with SES (n = 585), BMS (n = 483) or CABG (n = 483). Stenting and CABG resulted in improvement of HRQoL and anginal status. Patients treated with SES had, on average, 10% better HRQoL than BMS patients from the first month up to 3 years (better score in subscales: physical functioning, physical role functioning, emotional role functioning and mental health). Up to 12 months, the HRQoL was better after SES implantation than CABG, but was identical thereafter. Angina was more prevalent in the BMS group than in the SES and CABG groups. After 36 months, 10% of the patients treated with SES suffered from angina, aong with 13% of CABG patients and 20% of BMS patients. The authors claimed that stenting and CABG resulted in a significant improvement in HRQoL and angina. Moreover, with a substantial reduction of restenosis, HRQoL after the use of SES was improved significantly compared with BMS, and was similar to that for CABG [37].

Recently published data from the Synergy between PCI with Taxus and Cardiac Surgery (SYNTAX) study showed additional information concerning HRQoL in patients treated with PCI using DES and CABG. The SYNTAX study was a large (n = 1,800), randomized trial in which the outcomes of PCI with the use of PES were compared with those of CABG among patients with three-vessel or left main CAD. Among patients treated by surgeons the composite primary endpoint (death, MI, stroke or repeat revascularization) was lower than that in the PCI group, but no significant differences between the two strategies in the composite of irreversible outcomes (death, MI or stroke) were noted. Investigators in the SYNTAX study carried out a prospective QoL substudy as a part of the main trial. They used a disease-specific measure (the SAQ) and two generic measures (SF-36 and EQ-5D) before and 1, 6 and 12 months after the procedure. The scores on the subscales of both questionnaires were higher at 6 months and 12 months than at baseline in PCI and CABG groups. The proportion of patients who were free from angina in CABG and PCI groups was similar at 1 month and 6 months, but was higher in the CABG group at 12 months (76.3% versus 71.6%, p = 0.05). Scores on other subscales of the SAQ and SF-36 were slightly higher in the PCI group (especially at 1 month) or similar in both groups (at 12 month follow-up). According to the authors, symptomatic benefits of CABG were counterbalanced by the faster recovery and improved short-term health status in PCI group. Both strategies resulted in significant relief from angina and improvement in overall health status [38].

Steady progress is being made with respect to the different technical aspects of CABG. Endoscopic technology is being used in an increasing number of CABG procedures. Endoscopic cardiosurgery allows for greater improvement in HRQoL than "off-pump" procedures (without the use of external circulation) or conventional CABG. This is related to significantly decreased postoperative pain and an earlier return to everyday activities. No differences in HRQoL 6 months after off-pump and on-pump CABG have been reported [39]. It has also been demonstrated that total arterial (bilateral internal thoracic arteries) CABG is feasible and safe in terms of in-hospital mortality. At follow-up, the incidence of death, hospital readmission and reintervention, and patient QoL are acceptable, with favorable graft patency rates [40]. These impressive short- and medium-term results should be confirmed in further studies.

4.4 PCI in ACS

ACS include acute myocardial infarction (AMI; which can be non-ST elevation myocardial infarction (NSTEMI) or ST elevation myocardial infarction (STEMI)) and unstable angina. There has been a decrease in mortality and other cardiac events resulting from aggressive, invasive treatment of STEMI and NSTEMI. Unstable angina is the most common diagnosis in patients admitted to Cardiac Intensive Care Units, more common than STEMI.

Dias et al., analyzing the HRQoL of 278 patients admitted to hospital for ACS, found that men, younger individuals, smokers, and those with better education were characterized by higher HRQoL [41]. Using SF-36, they found significantly lower values for the Physical Component Summary (PCS) and Mental Component Summary (MCS) in individuals who previously experienced a cardiovascular incident and presented with symptoms of depression. A worse perception of physical health was more often encountered in patients with hypertension and DM who lived alone. No relationship was found between HRQoL and symptoms or complications due to hospitalization. Worse psychological health (lower MCS score on SF-36) was observed in long-term observation of women, a baseline MCS < 56 points, and in those with symptoms of depression. PCS values below the mean were also found in long-term observations of women as well as in patients with previous cardiovascular incidents, hypertension, DM, dyslipidemia, and a lower level of education. Patients with higher PCS values in long-term observation were usually smokers, typically had higher PCS and MCS values, and exhibited fewer symptoms of depression. PCI in ACS patients led to improvement in HRQoL. In logistic regression analyses, male sex, high baseline PCS, a higher level of education, and no previous cardiovascular incidents were independent predictors of good physical health after PCI. Conversely, female sex and symptoms of depression were independent predictors of worse MCS values [41].

The Fragmin and/or Early Revascularization During Instability in Coronary Artery Disease (FRISC II) study found that invasive treatment led to improvement in the HRQoL of 2,457 patients measured using SF-36 and the Angina Pectoris Quality of Life (APQLQ) questionnaire. Compared with the conservatively (pharmacologically) treated group, improvement was observed 12 months after the procedure [42]. The authors also confirmed that the presence and exacerbation of angina had a significant, detrimental influence on HRQoL in short- and long-term observation. Also, compared with healthy individuals, unstable angina pectoris significantly decreased the HRQoL of patients. This study expanded on the earlier results of the FRISC II study, which found decreased exacerbation of angina and exercise-based ischemia symptoms in patients referred for invasive therapy.

Invasive treatment of ACS leads to improvement in HRQoL by decreasing the degree and severity of angina symptoms. However, it is not known if the strategy of carrying out invasive interventions at an early stage leads to a significant improvement in HRQoL or if aggressive pharmacotherapy which reduces the symptoms of angina lead to improvement in HRQoL. The latter seems to be less likely, especially in the presence of advanced atherosclerotic changes responsible for coronary instability [1].

The Third Randomized Intervention Trial of Unstable Angina (RITA-3) compared the influence of using invasive therapy undertaken at an early stage or conservative therapy on the HRQoL of subjects with unstable angina or NSTEMI [43]. "Invasive treatment" referred to pharmacotherapy with early diagnostic coronography (including the possibility of revascularization), and "conservative treatment" referred to stabilizing symptoms using pharmacotherapy alone (with possible coronography should angina symptoms persist or hallmarks of cardiac ischemia appear). Treatment was randomly chosen for 1,810 patients, 895 of whom were treated invasively and 915 were treated conservatively. HRQoL was evaluated using a battery of tests administered at baseline and after 1 year follow-up: SF-36, SAQ, EQ-VAS, and EQ-5D. As measured by EQ-VAS and EQ-5D at 12 months, significant improvement in general HRQoL and self-rated heath status was found in the early invasively treated group compared with the conservatively treated group. In early invasively treated groups, an improvement in HRQoL at 12 months was observed also in SF-36 (i.e., better physical, emotional, and social functioning as well as greater vitality and better general health) and SAQ (i.e., higher scores for exercise tolerance, stabilized angina, satisfaction with treatment, and self-rated health status).

Primary angioplasty undertaken in patients with MI significantly decreases mortality. However, only a few authors have simultaneously examined survival and HRQoL in patients after STEMI. It is no doubt that older age is a risk factor for higher mortality after AMI. Ho et al. assessed a prospective cohort of 2,498 patients from the Prospective Registry Evaluating Outcomes After Myocardial Infarction: Events and Recovery Quality Improvement Registry (PREMIER) for HRQoL and burden of angina among survivors of MI in several age groups (> 75 years, 65–74 years, 50–64 years, and 19–49 years) using the SAQ [44]. Multivariable analyses assessed the relationship between age and 1-year HRQoL as well as angina burden, adjusting for differences in clinical characteristics, treatment and baseline health status. Older patients comprised a majority; 20.1% were aged ≥ 75 years, 41.7% were 65–74 years, 20.7% were 50–64 years, and 17.4% were < 50 years. At 12 months, older patients had a higher mortality (17.0% versus 8.7% versus 6.1% versus 3.2% for age groups ≥ 75, 65–74, 50–64, and 19–49 years, respectively, $p < 0.001$). Among survivors of AMI, increasing age was associated with fewer angina symptoms and better HRQoL. These findings revealed that older patients had the potential for successful functional recovery after AMI. However, 1 in 10 of the oldest patients and nearly 1 in 4 younger patients experienced angina 1 year after AMI. These data highlighted the importance of continued symptom surveillance after AMI, and suggested the need for better strategies to reduce symptom burden. The finding that older survivors of AMI had successful functional and symptomatic recovery after AMI despite receiving lower rates of some evidence-based therapies (such as invasive and EBM pharmacological treatment) suggests even greater benefits in HRQL may have been possible if guidelines were followed regardless of age. Those findings were also supported by Shah et al., who found that aggressive treatment of CAD patients older than 85 years was associated with prolongation of survival and improvement in QoL [45].

The possible influence of depression on the HRQoL in patients with ACS is also important. Thombs et al. investigated whether symptoms of depression during hospitalization for ACS, or the course of depressive symptoms after ACS, predict physical health status 12 months after ACS, after controlling for physical health status at the time of the ACS [46]. This was a prospective study of 425 patients with ACS assessed with the Beck Depression Inventory (BDI) and Short Form 12 (SF-12) Health Survey during hospitalization and 12 months later. Linear regression was used to assess the relationship between in-hospital BDI scores and BDI symptoms after ACS with physical health status 12 months later, after controlling for baseline physical health status, age, sex, Killip class, history of AMI, and the cardiac diagnosis. Baseline BDI scores predicted 12-month physical health. Compared with non-depressed patients, only patients with persistent symptoms of depression were at risk of poorer physical health. Patients with newly developed depressive symptoms after ACS were at slightly increased risk for worsened physical health, whereas patients with transient depressive symptoms were not at increased risk. These results underlined the importance of assessing depression at the time of ACS and on an ongoing basis. The authors did not supply information about the treatment (invasive or non-invasive) of patients.

Results from large studies suggest a role for psychosocial factors as prognostic factors in cardiovascular disease, with the strongest evidence for depression as a negative factor in post-infarction patients. However, whether depression is an independent risk (after adjustment for conventional risk factors) is unclear and there is little evidence that interventions targeting these factors improve the prognosis [47]. Data also suggest that self-reported measures of health status may predict mortality in ACS patients, and the brief SF-12 PCS can present an attractive option for improving risk stratification in ACS. In one of such studies, Thombs et al. administered the SF-12 and BDI to 800 ACS patients 2–5 days after admission to a Coronary Care Unit [48]. They used logistic regression to assess the relationship of the PCS and MCS with mortality 12 months later, after controlling for age, sex, cardiac diagnosis (MI versus unstable angina), Killip class, history of MI, and in-hospital depressive symptoms. Lower scores on the SF-12 PCS (worse health) were associated with a significantly higher risk of mortality, whereas MCS scores failed to reach significance. PCS significantly predicted mortality even after controlling for other cardiac risk factors and depressive symptoms, equivalent to a 34% increase in risk per 10-point (1 SD) decrement in PCS scores (see Appendix).

Comorbidities such as DM may also influence HRQoL in patients with ACS. Peterson et al. investigated a prospective cohort of 1,199 patients with ACS from whom 326 (37%) suffered from DM. Patients with DM were: more likely to present with unstable angina (52% versus 40%); less likely to present with STEMI (20% versus 31%); less likely to undergo coronary angiography (68% versus 82%). In multivariable analyses, DM was associated with significantly more angina, cardiac-related physical limitations, and HRQoL deficits at 1 year [49].

Patients suffering from cardiogenic shock in the course of ACS constitute a separate group. The Should we Emergently Evascularize Occluded Coronaries for Cardiogenic Shock (SHOCK) study found that emergency revascularization in patients with cardiogenic shock could reduce mortality in this group by 51% [50]. However, though cardiac damage preceding shock is usually diffuse, survivors may have to deal with secondary restrictions placed on their exercise tolerance and HRQoL. Sleeper et al. compared the HRQoL of patients 2 weeks after hospital discharge and 1 year after their intervention for cardiogenic shock [51]. They found that improvement in the HRQoL of patients who were randomly assigned to emergency revascularization was higher than in the group randomly assigned to conservative treatment. Also, fewer cases of congestive heart failure were noted in the PCI group. However, considering the small number of participants in this study, several questions (including the influence of age and sex on the HRQoL of individuals with cardiogenic shock) remain to be answered.

References

1. Hlatky MA (2004) Coronary revascularization and quality of life. Am Heart J 148:5-6
2. Bertuccio P, Levi F, Lucchini F et al (2011) Coronary heart disease and cerebrovascular disease mortality in young adults: recent trends in Europe. Eur J Cardiovasc Prev Rehabil 18:627-634
3. Rodríguez T, Malvezzi M, Chatenoud L et al (2006) Trends in mortality from coronary heart and cerebrovascular diseases in the Americas: 1970-2000. Heart 92:453-460
4. Mommersteeg PM, Denollet J, Spertus JA, Pedersen SS (2009) Health status as a risk factor in cardiovascular disease: a systematic review of current evidence. Am Heart J 157: 208-218
5. Xie J, Wu EQ, Zheng Z-J et al (2008) Patient-reported health status in coronary heart disease in the United States. Age, sex, racial and ethnic differences. Circulation 118:491-497
6. Wijns W, Kolh P, Danchin N et al (2010) Guidelines on myocardial revascularization. Task Force on Myocardial Revascularization of the European Society of Cardiology (ESC) and the European Association for Cardio-Thoracic Surgery (EACTS); European Association for Percutaneous Cardiovascular Interventions (EAPCI) Eur Heart J 31:2501-2555
7. Bucher HC, Hengstler P, Schindler C, Guyatt GH (2000) Percutaneous transluminal coronary angioplasty versus medical treatment for non-acute coronary heart disease: meta-analysis of randomised controlled trials. BMJ 321:73-77
8. Benzer W, Hofer S, Oldridge NB (2003) Health-related quality of life in patients with coronary artery disease after different treatments for angina in routine clinical practice. Herz 28:421-428
9. Westin L, Nilstun T, Carlsson R, Erhardt L (2005) Patients with ischemic heart disease: quality of life predicts long-term mortality. Scand Cardiovasc J 39:50-54
10. Folland ED, Hartigan PM, Parisi AF (1997) Percutaneous transluminal coronary angioplasty versus medical therapy for stable angina pectoris: outcomes for patients with double-vessel versus single-vessel coronary artery disease in a Vetrenas Affairs Cooperative randomized trial. Veterans Affairs ACME Investigators. J Am Coll Cardiol 29:1505-1511

11. Spertus JA, Salisbury AC, Jones PG et al (2004) Predictors of quality-of-life benefit after percutaneous coronary intervention. Circulation 110:3789-3794
12. Boden WE, O'Rourke RA, Teo KK et al (2007) Optimal medical therapy with or without PCI for stable coronary disease. N Engl J Med 35:1503-1516
13. Weintraub WS, Spertus JA, Kolm P et al (2008) Effect of PCI on quality of life in patients with stable coronary disease. N Engl J Med 359:677-687
14. Peterson ED, Rumsfeld JS (2008) Finding the Courage to reconsider medical therapy for stable angina. N Engl J Med 359:751-753
15. Holubkov R, Laskey WK, Haviland A et al (2002) Angina 1 year after percutaneous coronary intervention: a report from the NHLBI Dynamic registry. Am Heart J 144:826-833
16. Rihal CS, Raco DL, Gersh BJ, Yusuf S (2003) Indications for coronary artery bypass surgery and percutaneous coronary interventions in chronic stable angina: review of the evidence and methodological considerations. Circulation 108:2439-2455
17. Permanyer-Miralda G, Alonso J, Brotons C et al (1999) Perceived health over 3 years after percutaneous coronary balloon angioplasty. J Clin Epidemiol 52:615-623
18. Pocock SJ, Henderson RA, Seed A et al (1996) Quality of life, employment status, and anginal symptoms after coronary angioplasty or bypass surgery: 3-year follow-up in the Randomized Intervention Treatment of Angina (RITA) Trial. Circulation 94:135-142
19. Nash IS, Curtis LH, Rubin H (1999) Predictors of patient-reported physical and mental health 6 months after percutaneous coronary revascularization. Am Heart J 138:422-429
20. de Quadros AS, Lima TC, Rodrigues AP et al (2011) Quality of life and health status after percutaneous coronary intervention in stable angina patients: results from the real-world practice. Catheter Cardiovasc Interv 77:954-960
21. The TIME Investigators (2001) Trial of Invasive versus Medical Therapy in Elderly patients with chronic symptomatic coronary-artery disease (TIME): a randomized trial. Lancet 358:951-957
22. Buser MA, Buser PT, Kuster GM et al (2008) Improvements in physical and mental domains of quality of life by anti-ischaemic drug and revascularization treatment in elderly men and women with chronic angina. Heart 94:1413-1418
23. Henderson RA, Pocock SJ, Clayton TC et al (2003) Seven-year outcome in the RITA-2 trial trail: coronary angioplasty versus medical therapy. J Am Coll Cardiol 42:1161-1170
24. Pfisterer M for the TAIM Investigators (2004) Long-term outcome in elderly patients with chronic angina managed invasively versus by optimized medical therapy. Four-year follow-up of the Randomized Trial of Invasive versus Medical Therapy in Elderly Patients (TIME). Circulation 110:1213-1218
25. Seto TB, Taira DA, Berezin R et al (2000) Percutaneous coronary revascularization in elderly patients: impact on functional status and quality of life. Ann Intern Med 132:955-958
26. Li R, Yan BP, Dong M et al (2012) Quality of life after percutaneous coronary intervention in the elderly with acute coronary syndrome. Int J Cardiol 155:90-96
27. Schenkeveld L, Pedersen SS, Nierop JWI et al (2010) Health-related quality of life and long-term mortality in patients treated with percutaneous coronary intervention. Am Heart J 159:471-476
28. Pedersen SS, Versteeg H, Denollet J et al (2011) Patient-rated health status predicts prognosis following percutaneous coronary intervention with drug-eluting stentiong. Qual Life Res 20:559-567
29. Park D-W, Yun S-C, Lee S-W et al (2008) Long-term mortality after percutaneous coronary intervention with drug-eluting stent implantation versus coronary artery bypass surgery for the treatment of multivessel coronary artery disease. Circulation 117:2079-2086
30. Hlatky MA, Boothroyd DB, Melsop KA et al (2004) Medical costs and quality of life 10 to 12 years after randomization to angioplasty or bypass surgery for multivessel coronary artery disease. Circulation 110:1960-1966
31. Zhang Z, Mahoney EM, Stables RH et al (2003) Disease-specific health status following stent-assisted percutaneous coronary intervention and coronary artery bypass surgery: 1-year results from the Stent or Surgery trial. Circulation 108:1694-1700

32. Favarato ME, Hueb W, Boden WE et al (2007) Quality of life in patients with symptomatic multivessel coronary artery disease: a comparative post hoc analyses of medical, angioplasty or surgical strategies-MASS II trial. Intern J Cardiol 116:364-370
33. Serruys PW, Unger F, Sousa E et al (2001) Comparison of coronary-artery-bypass surgery and stenting for the treatment of multivessel disease. N Engl J Med 344:1117-1124
34. Zhang Z, Weintraub WS, Mahoney EM et al (2004) Relative benefit of coronary artery bypass grafting versus stent-assisted percutaneous coronary intervention for angina pectoris and multivessel coronary artery disease in women versus men (one-year results from the Stent or Surgery Trial). Am J Cardiol 93:404-409
35. Serruys PW, Ong ATL, Morice M-C et al (2005) Arterial Revascularisation Therapies Study Part II – sirolimus-eluting stents for the treatment of patients with multivessel de novo coronary artery lesions. EuroIntervention 1:147-156
36. Daemen J, Kuck KH, Macaya C et al (2008) Multivessel coronary revascularization in patients with and without diabetes mellitus. J Am Coll Cardiol 52:1957-1967
37. van Domburg RT, Daemen J, Morice MC et al (2010) Short- and long-term health related quality-of-life and anginal status of the Arterial Revascularisation Therapies Study part II, ARTS-II; sirolimus-eluting stents for the treatment of patients with multivessel coronary artery disease. Euro Intervention 5:962-967
38. Cohen DJ, Van Hout B, Serruys PW et al (2011) Synergy between PCI with Taxus and Car diac Surgery Investigators. Quality of life after PCI with drug-eluting stents or coronary-artery bypass surgery. N Engl J Med 364:1016-1026
39. Kapetanakis EI, Stamou SC, Petro KR et al (2008) Comparison of the quality of life after conventional versus off-pump coronary artery bypass surgery. J Card Surg 23:120-125
40. Navia D, Vrancic M, Vaccarino G et al (2008) Total arterial off-pump coronary revascularization using bilateral thoracic arteries in triple-vessel disease: surgical technique and clinical outcomes. Ann Thorac Surg 86:524-530
41. Dias CC, Mateus P, Santos L et al (2005) Acute coronary syndrome and predictors of quality of life. Rev Port Cardiol 24:819-831
42. Janzon M, Levin LA, Swahn E (2004) Invasive treatment in unstable coronary artery disease promotes health-related quality of life: results from the FRISC II trial. Am Heart J 148:112-119
43. Kim J, Henderson RA, Pocock SJ et al (2005) Health-related quality of life after inteventional or conservative strategy in patients with unstable angina or non-ST-segment elevation myocardial infarction. One-year results of the Third Randomized Intervention Trial of Unstable Angina (RITA-3). J Am Coll Cardiol 45:221-228
44. Ho MP, Eng MH, Rumsfeld JS et al (2008) The influence of age on health status outcomes after acute myocardial infarction. Am Heart J 155:855-861
45. Shah P, Najafi AH, Panza JA et al (2009) Outcomes and quality of life in patients ≥ 85 years of age with ST-elevation myocardial infarction. Am J Cardiol 103:170-174
46. Thombs BD, Ziegelstein RC, Stewart DE et al (2008) Usefulness of persistent symptoms of depression to predict physical health status 12 months after an acute coronary syndrome. Am J Cardiol 101:15-19
47. Van de Werf F, Bax J, Betriu A et al (2008) Management of acute myocardial infarction in patients presenting with persistent ST-segment elevation. Eur Heart J 29:2909-2945
48. Thombs BD, Ziegelstein RC, Stewart DE et al (2008) Physical health status assessed during hospitalization for acute coronary syndrome predicts mortality 12 month later. J Psychosom Res 65:587-593
49. Peterson PN, Spertus JA, Magid JD et al (2006) The impact of diabetes on one-year health status outcomes following acute coronary syndromes. BMC Cardiovasc Dis 6:41
50. Hochman JS, Sleeper LA, White HD et al (2001) One-year survival following early revascularization for cardiogenic shock. JAMA 285:190-192
51. Sleeper LA, Ramanathan K, Picard MH et al (2005) Functional status and quality of life after emergency revascularization for cardiogenic shock complicating acute myocardial infarction. J Am Coll Cardiol 46:266-273

5 Quality of Life in Patients with Chronic Heart Failure

Marek Klocek and Danuta Czarnecka

5.1 Introduction

Despite advances in treatment leading to prolongation of survival, chronic heart failure (CHF) remains the primary cause of death among individuals with cardiovascular diseases (CVDs) [1]. Heart failure is associated with heavy symptom burden, frequent admission into hospital, and high mortality. The incidence of CHF increases with age, and the prognosis is similar to the prevalence of mortality seen in certain malignant neoplasms [2]. Data from the West Midlands Regional Cancer Registry in the UK found that the 1-year survival of CHF patients was worse than that of patients with cancers of the breast, prostate gland, or bladder [3].

Symptomatic heart failure negatively influences the quality of life (QoL) of subjects by restricting various spheres of activity and social role functioning. Individuals with heart failure usually experience high levels of physical, functional and emotional distress, and their health-related quality of life (HRQoL) cannot be normalized even with optimal treatment [4, 5]. The QoL of patients with heart failure and their partners is poor compared with: (i) their age-matched peers from the general population; (ii) patients suffering from other chronic diseases. Moreover, depression is a strong determinant of the QoL of CHF patients [6]. It has been demonstrated that male patients complain about significant fatigue, a lack of energy, and a resigned demeanor [7]. Conversely, women are characterized by increased perception of all the negative symptoms of CHF: they lose trust in themselves, worry, and feel a heightened sense of anxiety [8]. These attitudes add to an increased dependence on their surroundings and negatively affect family life [9]. The psychological state of subjects, independent of the symptoms of CHF, leads to more frequent and extended hospitalization.

M. Klocek (✉)
I Department of Cardiology and Hypertension
Jagiellonian University Medical College, Kraków, Poland
e-mail: marek.klocek@wp.pl

K. Kawecka-Jaszcz et al. (eds.), *Health-Related Quality of Life in Cardiovascular Patients*,
DOI: 10.1007/978-88-470-2769-5_5

In recent years, interest has focused on the HRQoL of CHF patients, which has since become an important endpoint in assessing the effects of different treatment options. However, when using the concept of HRQoL, one should be mindful that it does not equate to "health status". Current health status is one of the determinants of HRQoL but, in actuality, it is a concept used to consider only a clinical understanding of health. A physician is interested initially in the changes to the biochemical and physiologic parameters under treatment. However, patients are more interested in alleviating symptoms, improving everyday functioning, and fulfilling their social roles. For patients, QoL (e.g., symptoms and the impact of their illness on social, emotional and occupational functioning) may be as important as longevity [10]. Because it offers information concerning the patient's experience of treatment, measuring HRQoL is a useful and significant expansion of traditional, clinical medicine, which measures health status based on the results of physical examination or laboratory results [11].

HRQoL is also a valuable prognostic indicator. For patients in the same CHF functional class (for example, a class set by the New York Heart Association (NYHA)), those with low HRQoL are characterized by a significantly greater risk of hospitalization related to their underlying disease, including a higher risk of mortality [12]. Rodriguez-Artalejo et al. [13] found that poor HRQoL in patients first hospitalized for heart failure measured using physical, psychological, and general health dimensions was associated with a 63–75% higher risk of rehospitalization and mortality within 6 months. Thus, treatment and care should focus not only on the physical symptoms of heart failure, but also on a multidisciplinary care approach involving optimizing medical therapy, symptom management, education, and the interventions known to improve QoL.

The main symptoms of CHF restricting everyday activity and leading to decreased HRQoL include dyspnea, fatigue, weakness, limited exercise tolerance, drowsiness, and peripheral edema. The HRQoL of CHF patients is significantly worse compared with that of healthy individuals or even those suffering from other chronic diseases (e.g., hypertension, diabetes mellitus (DM), atrial fibrillation, angina, post-myocardial infarction, or chronic obstructive pulmonary disease (COPD)) [4, 14]. CHF patients suffer from limited exercise tolerance, which inhibits an active lifestyle. However, it has long been observed that evaluation of traditional clinical endpoints (e.g., physician-rated exercise tolerance, left ventricular ejection fraction, concentration of N-terminal prohormone of brain natriuretic peptide (NT-proBNP) in blood) correlate poorly (if at all) with the degree of everyday activity and general wellbeing of CHF patients [6] who, in similar stages of clinical advancement, function and react differently in various, everyday life situations. HRQoL could be (and usually is) impaired in heart-failure patients with preserved and reduced left ventricular ejection fraction (LVEF) [15].

Personal relationships, nutrition, sexual activity, and the ability to work are restricted in heart-failure patients and coalesce with an increasing dependency upon others. HRQoL is determined not by the fact that these problems and difficulties are present, but by the manner in which they are dealt with, experienced, and how the patient responds to these events. Differences in how patients interpret their situation during the course of illness may lead to reductions in everyday functioning and social relationships, resulting in constrained social support. Conversely, the inability of family and one's surroundings to accommodate the illness-related needs of a close individual (i.e., ineffective support) leads to restrictions placed on contact with the patient, further decreasing HRQoL. The partners of CHF patients have also been found to report decreased HRQoL [16]. A worsening health status reminds the patient of impending death, leading to worsened psychosocial health (i.e., depression, increased anxiety and sleep disturbances) [6]. HRQoL therefore remains a significant problem for CHF patients and their families. "Objective health status", in the traditional, medical sense of the term, constitutes only a part of this problem.

5.2 Measuring HRQoL in Subjects with CHF

Measuring QoL (including measurements in CHF patients) is usually realized by the use of two types of questionnaire: generic and specific. Their application is meant to illustrate and describe the consequences of illness from the patient's perspective. The generic instruments most often used in heart-failure patients are the Psychological General Wellbeing (PGWB) Index, the Life Satisfaction Questionnaire, the Nottingham Health Profile (NHP), the Sickness Impact Profile (SIP) and the Short Form Health Survey 36 (SF-36) (see Appendix). Several specific questionnaires can also be applied to CHF patients. These can be used to measure HRQoL or measure selected dimensions of QoL (Table 5.1).

Specific questionnaires are usually less broad than the generic questionnaires, and allow for better understanding of how treatment influences a specific problem, such as symptoms, physical activity, and sexual dysfunction. The specific questionnaires most often used in CHF patients are the Quality of Life in Severe Heart Failure Questionnaire (QLQ-SHF), the Chronic Heart Failure Questionnaire (CHFQ), the Kansas City Cardiomyopathy Questionnaire (KCCQ), the Left Ventricular Dysfunction Questionnaire (LVD-36), the Minnesota Living with Heart Failure Questionnaire (MLHF), and the European Heart Failure Self-Care Behavior Scale [17, 18]. These questionnaires have good psychometric properties (validity and sensitivity to change), though in patients suffering from CHF current evidence would primarily support the use of the MLHF, followed by the KCCQ and CHFQ.

The MLHF has been applied in research such as the Studies of Left Ventricular

Table 5.1 Questionnaires used to measure health-related quality of life in subjects with chronic heart failure (see Appendix)

Generic	Chronic heart failure-specific or targeted	Domain or factor-specific
Short Form Health Survey 36 (SF-36)	Minnesota Living with Heart Failure (MLHF)	Hospital Anxiety Depression Scale (HADS)
Sickness Impact Profile (SIP)	Chronic Heart Failure Questionnaire (CHFQ)	Duke Activity Status Index (DASI)
Dortmund COOP Scale (COOP)	QoL in Severe Heart Failure Questionnaire (QLQ-SHF)	Reitan Trail-making Test
EuroQoL 5D (EQ-5D)	Subjective Symptoms Assessment Profile (SSA-P)	Six-minute Walking Test (6MWT)
Nottingham Health Profile (NHP)	Heart Failure Functional Status Inventory (HFFSI)	Katz Index of Activities of Daily Living (KIAD)
Psychological General Wellbeing Index (PGWB)	MacNew Questionnaire (MacNew)	International Index of Erectile Dysfunction (IIEF-5)
Quality of Life Index (QLI)	European Heart Failure Self-Care Behaviour Scale	Profiles of Mood States (POMS)
The Self Assessment of Global Wellbeing (SAGWB)	QoL in Severe Heart Failure Questionnaire (QLQ-SHF)	
WHO Quality of Life Questionnaire (WHOQoL)	Kansas City Cardiomyopathy Questionnaire (KCCQ)	
Cantril Ladder of Life (CLL)	Left Ventricular Dysfunction Questionnaire (LVD-36)	

Dysfunction, Vasodilator-Heart Failure Trials (V-HeFT II and III), and to measure the results of using different beta-blockers in the treatment of heart failure. A randomized study comparing the influence of digoxin and placebo on HRQoL was done using the CHFQ. Also, the QLQ-SHF was used in various studies examining how the course of CHF is influenced by the use of angiotensin-converting enzyme inhibitors (ACEIs). Further discussion is required regarding the use of specific questionnaires applied in the measurement of HRQoL in patients with heart failure (see Appendix).

5.2.1 QLQ-SHF

QLQ-SHF comprises 26 Likert-type questions used to measure quantitatively physical activity as well as an analogous scale to measure life satisfaction and social/emotional factors. The higher the point score, the more negatively affected is HRQoL. QLQ-SHF has been used in several clinical studies, and its validity has been determined in comparative studies with other questionnaires (e.g., SIP). The validity of the QLQ-SHF is sufficient for the dimensions of physical symptoms and life satisfaction. However, this validity is decreased for somatic complaints and physical activity.

Studies have shown that the QLQ-SHF is moderately sensitive to small changes in the QoL of CHF patients. However, further study is required because it is not known if this questionnaire can be used to differentiate between patients in terms of CHF severity (see Appendix).

5.2.2 CHFQ

CHFQ contains 20 questions which can be applied in an interview with trained personnel. It can be used to differentiate between three problem categories: dyspnea, fatigue, and emotional functioning. A higher score denotes higher HRQoL. CHFQ is highly sensitive to changes in the degree of severity of the main CHF symptoms (i.e., dyspnea and fatigue). Therefore, CHFQ is used in patients at varying levels of CHF advancement (see Appendix).

5.2.3 MLHF

MLHF was developed for CHF patients to measure how such patients interpret the influence of CHF on their exercise tolerance, socioeconomic functioning, and psychological status (see Appendix). Patients answer 21 questions using a six-level, Likert-type scale, earning 0–5 points for each answer. One can measure the dimensions of physical and emotional functioning separately. MLHF is short, easy to use, and understandable by patients. It can be administered as a survey and completely independently by patients in their homes or in the physician's office. MLHF has satisfactory validity compared with other scales measuring the influence of CHF on the HRQoL of patients [19].

It can be used to differentiate between subjects with and without symptomatic left ventricular dysfunction (LVD) (i.e., NYHA classes I and II) but it poorly differentiates between advanced stages of symptomatic CHF. Thers are reservations as to whether MLHF can also be used to differentiate between symptoms of heart failure from similar symptoms in other diseases [20]. MLHF is usually employed to measure heart-related QoL in CHF patients, but it is a specific questionnaire that is meant to be used in clinical studies to measure the influence of pharmacotherapy or other interventions on HRQoL. It does not ensure a full measure of HRQoL [20].

5.3 Clinical Factors and the HRQoL of CHF Patients

Burdensome symptoms reported by 20–75% of heart-failure patients include dyspnea, fatigue, pain, peripheral edema, and lack of appetite. Beyond these typical symptoms of failing health, ≤ 70% of CHF patients experience anxiety and 50% report depressive symptoms, excessive stress, and cognitive dysfunction (i.e., difficulty with concentration). Approximately 50% of patients also experience dry mouth, trouble with taste sensations, excessive sweating, palpitations, and constipation [21].

Dyspnea and fatigue are the basic symptoms reported by CHF patients. Patients also complain about sleep disturbances, described by them as "even worse and more burdensome" than dyspnea [21], leading to even greater fatigue and negative influences on HRQoL [22]. A significant percentage of CHF patients report aggravated sleep disturbances, especially insomnia. These disturbances are associated directly not only with fatigue, but also the frequent occurrence of depression and poor HRQoL [22]. It seems that CHF patients who report chronic fatigue along with tiredness during the day should also be evaluated carefully for sleep disturbances [23].

Worse HRQoL has been linked to a younger age of the CHF patient, greater severity of symptoms, and to a greater number of restrictions on physical activity resulting from CHF [21]. Decreasing the severity or eliminating the symptoms of CHF leads to an improved ability to engage in normal activity and may positively influence HRQoL. Most CHF patients know that their illness is related to reduced longevity, which leads to additional stress.

Female CHF patients are characterized by having lower HRQoL than men [24]. Their HRQoL is also lower than that of women who have experienced a myocardial infarction (MI) or in those with other chronic diseases, such as DM, Parkinson's disease, or COPD [25]. Compared with men, the HRQoL of female CHF patients is most affected in the dimensions of: sleep; symptoms; the energy that they have every day; physical and psychological functioning; and self-rated health. Improvement in HRQoL after hospitalization due to CHF is also lower in women than in men.

Not all studies confirm the decreased HRQoL of women with heart failure. Compared with women, some authors observe decreased HRQoL in male subjects with heart failure, especially in older age groups [4, 26]. However, these differences disappeared after adjusting for the NYHA classification system, ejection fraction, and age. When explaining differences in the HRQoL of male and female subjects with CHF, the different ways in which the sexes perceive the influence of their disease on everyday functioning must be stated. Men tend to focus most of their attention on the restrictions their disease places on physical functioning. Conversely, women tend to focus their attention on the negative affects of their disease on emotional, family and social functioning. Women with poor social support, who live alone, and who have a pessimistic personality are characterized by especially lower HRQoL [27].

Congestive heart failure is one of the diseases that affects HRQoL most negatively, in which older (compared with younger) patients seem to report higher levels of QoL [22, 24, 26]. This difference is based primarily on the varied way in which health and illness is interpreted at different ages. Younger individuals are affected more greatly by the restrictions placed on them by their illness, even if this involves only their family and professional activities. Sexual dysfunction constitutes an often encountered problem in male CHF patients. This involves loss of libido and an increased incidence of erectile dysfunction [28].

Ejection fraction does not correlate significantly with HRQoL in CHF patients. Austin et al. reported that, at 8 years follow-up in patients living with heart failure, HRQoL scores were similar regardless of systolic function (i.e., the KCCQ scores were not different in the survivors with preserved and reduced ejection fraction) [29]. Recently, Hoekstra et al. confirmed that QoL measured with generic and diseases-specific questionnaires was impaired by similar amounts in CHF patients with preserved ejection fraction as in CHF patients with reduced ejection fraction [15].

5.4 Influence of Treatment for Heart Failure on HRQoL

Studies have shown that pharmacological and non-pharmacological (e.g., restricting intake of salt and fluids) treatment options may positively influence the HRQoL of CHF patients (though this effect is not appreciable). In patients with symptomatic left ventricular dysfunction, certain ACEIs, beta-blockers (especially carvedilol) [30], and diuretics yield only a modest advantage over placebo in terms of improving HRQoL. In this respect, differences exist within groups of particular drugs. For example, compared with placebo, one study did not find rampril to significantly improve the HRQoL of patients treated for moderately advanced CHF.

Certain angiotensin-II receptor antagonists called sartans are characterized by their positive influence on the HRQoL of subjects with heart failure as measured using the McMaster questionnaire. The recently published results of the Candesartan in Heart Failure (CHARM) study [31] reported that, after 26 months, the addition of candesartan to current CHF treatment led to significant improvement in HRQoL. Moreover, the Valsartan Heart Failure Trial (Val-HeFT) found that adding valsartan to an ACEI regimen that did not include beta-blockers led to improvement in HRQoL if measured using MLHF [32]. Both studies suggested that, from the viewpoint of patient QoL, sartans may be used in CHF patients already being treated with ACEIs, or even before beginning treatment with beta-blockers.

However, not all studies have confirmed the additional benefits of sartan use on the HRQoL of heart-failure patients. The Losartan Heart Failure Survival Study

(ELITE II) measured HRQoL in CHF patients treated with losartan. It found that losartan did not have an advantage over captopril in terms of influencing the QoL of patients in NYHA classes II–IV and decreased left ventricular ejection fraction. The Replacement of Angiotensin Converting Enzyme Inhibition (REPLACE) study also did not find changes to the HRQoL of patients with heart failure treated with telmisartan compared with those treated with enalapril if measured using MLHF [33].

The dimensions most sensitive to pharmacological therapy include the symptoms of CHF and exercise tolerance. Changes to HRQoL influenced by pharmacological treatment are minimal or absent after the administration of drugs that are similar in their clinical effects and side effects. For example, of 10 studies examining the influence of beta-blockers on the HRQoL of patients with heart failure, only 3 reported improvement [34]. A study by Baxter et al. [35] found only modest improvement in general QoL and decreased severity of depression and anxiety if bisoprolol was used in CHF patients aged ≥ 70 years. Also, as part of a prospective study, a direct comparison of carvedilol and metoprolol found that they influenced the HRQoL of CHF patients in a similar way, despite certain hemodynamic differences favoring carvedilol [36]. Even with the use of new-generation beta-blockers (e.g., carvedilol, nebivolol), heart failure inevitably decreases the longevity and wellbeing of patients [37, 38].

Several drugs used to treat subjects with heart failure can reduce heart rate (HR), but their effects on symptoms are diverse and can be undesirable. Results from the Systolic Heart Failure Treatment with the If Inhibitor Ivabradine Trial (SHIFT) showed that HR reduction with ivabradine in CHF patients reduced cardiovascular mortality or hospital admissions for worsening heart failure. In addition, there was an improvement in NYHA class and in patient-reported QoL measured using the KCCQ [39]. HRQoL at follow-up was better preserved in the ivabradine group compared with placebo (ivabradine reduced HR by 10 bpm versus placebo). This study suggested that the ivabradine-associated reduction in CHF severity (as reflected by a reduced number of hospital admissions and improved NYHA functional class) also translated into a favorable impact on HRQoL. In contrast, treatment with beta-blockers (which were associated with similar HR reduction and reduction in CHF mortality) did not result in improved HRQoL, as reported in a meta-analysis by Dobre et al. [40].

Volterrani et al. found in the Effect of Carvedilol, Ivabradine or their Combination on Exercise Capacity in Patients with Heart Failure (CARVIVA HF) Trial that patients with heart failure treated with a maximal dose of ACEI who then received ivabradine or ivabradine plus carvedilol had better QoL than patients treated only with carvedilol. HR in this relatively small study (n = 121) was reduced in all three groups, but to a graeter extent by the combination [41]. The studies described above suggest that ivabradine alone or in combination with some beta-blockers may be effective in improving exercise tolerance and QoL in CHF patients.

How non-pharmacologic interventions influence HRQoL is even less conclusive. The results of recently published studies concerning different treatment options, beginning from basic nursing and ending with nasal continuous positive airway pressure (NCPAP), noted only a small positive influence of these interventions on the HRQoL of CHF patients. Patient education and regular support from nursing personnel seems to improve the HRQoL of patients at various stages of advanced heart failure [42].

Another problem in CHF patients is anemia, which is caused mainly by iron deficiency. Anemia is a strong risk factor for increased mortality in patients with CVDs (including CHF) and may be considered to be the biological background for one frequently reported complaint: chronic fatigue. Conversely, some CHF patients have iron deficiency without anemia. Beyond erythropoesis, iron is involved in many biological processes crucial for the maintenance of homeostasis. Its deficiency may impair the aerobic and oxidative metabolism of cells, leading to limitation in exercise capacity, decreased wellbeing and a poor prognosis in CHF patients [43]. The Ferinject Assessment in Patients with Iron Deficiency and Chronic Heart Failure (FAIR-HF) Trial [44] demonstrated that intravenous administration of ferric carboxymaltose in patients with CHF and iron deficiency with and without anemia could improve exercise performance and QoL in ≈50% of these patients as compared with 28% patients receiving placebo.

5.5 Influence of Physical Exercise on the HRQoL of CHF Patients

There is a direct relationship between CHF and worsened exercise tolerance resulting from a lack of physical training. Exercise improves the HRQoL of patients through benefits to their general physical condition and the possibility of independent functioning. The first randomized clinical study measuring the influence of physical training on patients with chronic CHF found that subjects, in general, felt better, more self-reliant, and had better control over their lives through participation in everyday activities with greater independence and less awareness of their illness [45].

Physical training in patients with heart failure usually involves the use of large muscle groups as well as strength exercises in small (i.e., peripheral) muscle groups. Training of large muscle groups consists of walking, step training, and ergometer cycling. Strength training in small muscle groups comprises exercises using arms or legs while sitting or lying down. It was recently observed that concentrated leg exercises (i.e., physical training of knee muscles), carried out over 8 weeks, led, in general, to improved exercise tolerance and improved HRQoL. This improvement was greater in the group training both legs as opposed to the group training only one leg. Therefore, the HRQoL of patients may (at least in part) be dependent upon the type of exercises done. Tyni-Lenne, et al. [46] conducted a study directly comparing changes in HRQoL resulting from the strength training of small muscle groups and ergometer cycling for large muscle groups. Improvement in HRQoL was noted only in patients who underwent small-muscle training of the lower limbs. This finding suggested that such training may be beneficial for subjects with more advanced CHF who are not very physically active, and that training small-muscle groups may correct the negative changes which occur in the peripheral muscles of CHF patients.

Studies examining the HRQoL of CHF patients subjected to physical training usually involve small patient groups who are typically middle-aged and therefore not representative of all patients with heart failure. Nevertheless, the vast majority of studies reported significant recovery in different dimensions of HRQoL in male and female subjects with CHF. Improving the HRQoL of heart-failure patients undergoing physical training is one of the most elusive elements of clinical improvement. Progress is associated with enhanced exercise tolerance, decreased fatigue and dyspnea, and an expansion in the everyday activity of patients (including an emotional dimension) [47]. Gradually increasing the resistance of weekly ergometer cycling is safe for CHF patients, and significantly develops their HRQoL as well as oxygen consumption, more so than training at a constant level of resistance [48]. Another study confirmed that gradually increasing the intensity of physical training improved HRQoL more so than less intensive training [49]. However, the long-term effects of such training on HRQoL remain to be determined; one study found a return to pre-training HRQoL levels 6 months after halting the exercise regimen [47].

Based on the studies mentioned above, supervised physical training of varied intensity may be advantageous for individuals with stable CHF in whom significant improvement in HRQoL occurs regardless of NYHA class or LVEF [45]. Physical training in older patients with exacerbated CHF symptoms leads to less improvement in HRQoL than in younger patients [50].

5.6 Conclusions

In CHF patients, HRQoL is worse than in patients suffering from other chronic diseases. Heart failure is associated with a heavy symptom burden, frequent hospitalization and high mortality. Many CHF patients are conscious of the fact that their illness is related to decreased longevity, which leads to added stress. They also suffer from chronic fatigue, depression, anxiety and sleep disturbances. QoL measured using appropriate questionnaires is also impaired in CHF patients with preserved ejection fraction as it is in those with reduced ejection fraction. However, contemporary pharmacotherapy, based mainly on ACEIs, sartans and beta-blockers, has a small (but beneficial) influence on symptoms and HRQoL. Moreover, patient education, support from nursing personnel, and regular physical training seem to improve the HRQoL of patients at various stages of heart failure.

References

1. Dickstein K, Cohen-Solal A, Filipatos G et al (2008) ESC Guidelines for the diagnosis and treatment of acute and chronic heart failure 2008. Eur Heart J 29:2388-2442
2. Stewart S, MacIntyre K, Hole DA et al (2000) More malignant than cancer? Five year survival following a first admission for heart failure in Scotland. Eur J Heart Fail 102:1126-1131
3. Cowie M, Kirby M (2001) Heart failure: an overview. Managing heart failure in primary care: a practical guide. Oxfordshire, UK, Bladon Medical Publishing, pp 1-5
4. Hobbs FDR, Kenkre JE, Roalfe AK et al (2002) Impact of heart failure and left ventricular systolic dysfunction on quality of life. Eur Heart J 23:1867-1876
5. Bekelman DB, Havranek EP, Becker DM et al (2007) Symptoms, depression, and quality of life in patients with heart failure. J Card Fail 13:643-648
6. Müller-Tasch T, Peters-Klimm F, Schellberg D et al (2007) Depression is a major determinant of quality of life in patients with chronic systolic heart failure in general practice. J Card Fail 13:818-824
7. Martensson J, Karlsson J-E, Friedlund B (1997) Male patients with congestive heart failure and their conception of life situation. J Adv Nures 25:579-586
8. Martensson J, Karlsson J-E, Friedlund B (1998) Female patients with congestive heart failure: how they conceive their life situation. J Adv Nures 28:1216-1224
9. Jaarsma T, Johansson P, Agren S et al (2010) Quality of life and symptoms of depression in advanced heart failure patients and their partners. Curr Opin Support Palliat Care 4:233-237
10. Stanek EJ, Oates MB, McGhanWF et al (2000) Preferences for treatment outcomes in patients with heart failure: symptoms vs. survival. J Card Fail 6:225-232
11. Johansson P, Agnebrink M, Dahlstrom U et al (2004) Measurement of health-related quality of life in chronic heart failure from a nursing perspective - a review of the literature. Eur J Cardiovasc Nurs 3:7-20
12. Alla F, Briancon S, Guillemin F et al (2002) Self-rating of quality of life provides additional prognostic information in heart failure. Insight into the EPICAL study. Eur J Heart Fail 4:337-343
13. Rodriguez-Artalejo F, Guallar-Castillon P, Pascual CR et al (2005) Health-related quality of life as a predictor of hospital readmission and death among patients with heart failure. Arch Intern Med 165:1274-1279
14. Juenger J, Schellberg D, Kraemer SH et al (2002) Health-related quality of life in patients with congestive heart failure: compared with other chronic diseases and relation to functional variables. Heart 87:235-241
15. Hoekstra T, Lesman-Leegte I, van Veldhuisen DJ et al (2011) Quality of life is impaired similarly in heart failure patients with preserved and reduced ejection fraction. Eur J Heart Fail 13:1013-1018
16. Luttik ML, Jaarsma T, Veeger NJ et al (2005) For better and for worse: Quality of life impaired in HF patients as well as in their partners. Eur J Cardiovasc Nurs 4:11-14
17. Jaarsma T, Stromberg A, Martensson J et al (2003) Development and testing of the European Heart Failure Self-Care Behaviour Scale. Eur J Heart Fail 5:363-370
18. Garin O, Ferrer M, Pont A et al (2009) Disease-specific health-related quality of life questionnaires for heart failure: a systematic review with meta-analyses. Qual Life Res 18:71-85
19. Hak T, Willems D, van der Wal G et al (2004) A qualitative validation of the Minnesota Living with Heart Failure Questionnaire. Qual Life Res 13:417-426
20. Sneed N, Paul S, Michel Y et al (2001) Evaluation of 3 quality of life measurement tools in patients with chronic heart failure. Heart Lung 30:332-340

21. Zambroski CH, Moser DK, Bhat G et al (2005) Impact of symptom prevalence and symptom burden on quality of life in patients with heart failure. Eur J Cardiovasc Nurs 4:198-206
22. Brostrom A, Stromberg A, Dahstrom U et al (2004) Sleep difficulties, daytime sleepness and health-related quality of life in patients with chronic heart failure. J Cardiovasc Nurs 4:234-242
23. Johansson P, Dahlstrom U, Brostrom A (2006) Factors and interventions influencing health-related quality of life in patients with heart failure: a review of the literature. Eur J Cardivasc Nurs 5:5-15
24. Steptoe A, Mohabir A, Mahon NG et al (2000) Health-related quality of life and psychological well-being in patients with dilated cardiomyopathy. Heart 83:645-650
25. Riedinger MS, Dracup KA, Brecht ML (2002) Studies of left ventricular dysfunction. Quality of life in women with heart failure, normative groups, and patients with other chronic conditions. Am J Critical Care 11:211-219
26. Ekman I, Fagerberg B, Lundman B (2002) Health-related quality of life and sense of coherence among elderly patients with severe chronic heart failure in comparison with healthy control. Heart Lung 31:94-101
27. Luttik ML, Jaarsma T, Veeger N et al (2006) Marital status, quality of life, and clinical outcome in patients with heart failure. Heart Lung 35:3-8
28. Jaarsma T (2002) Sexual problems in heart failure patients. Eur J Cardiovasc Nurs 1:61-67
29. Austin BA, Wang Y, Smith GL et al (2008) Systolic function as a predictor of mortality and quality of life in long-term survivors with heart failure. Clin Cardiol 31:119-124
30. Rickli H, Steiner S, Muller K et al (2004) Beta-blockers in heart failure: Carvedilol Safety Assessment (CASA 2-trial). Eur J Heart Fail 6:761-768
31. O'Meara E, Lewis E, Granger C et al (2005) Patient perception of the effect of treatment with candesartan in heart failure. Results of the Candesartan in Heart failure: Assessment of Reduction in Mortality and morbidity (CHARM) programme. Eur J Heart Fail 7:650-656
32. Krum H, Carson P, Farsang C et al (2004) Effect of valsartan added to background ACE inhibitor therapy in patients with heart failure: results from Val-HeFT. Eur J Heart Fail 6:937-945
33. Dunselman PH (2001) Effects of the replacement of the angiotensin converting enzyme inhibitor enalapril by the angiotensin II receptor blocker telmisartan in patients with congestive heart failure. The replacement of angiotensin converting enzyme inhibition (REPLACE) investigators. Intern J Cardiol 77:131-138
34. Reddy P, Dunn AB (2000) The effect of beta-blockers on health-related quality of life in patients with heart failure. Pharmacotherapy 20:679-689
35. Baxter AJ, Spensley A, Hildreth A et al (2002) Beta blockers in older persons with heart failure: tolerability and impact on quality of life. Heart 88:611-614
36. Metra M, Giubbini R, Nodari S et al (2000) Differential effects of beta-blockers in patients with heart failure: A prospective, randomized, double-blind comparison of the long-term effects of metoprolol versus carvedilol. Circulation 102:546-551
37. Cleland JG, Charlesworth A, Lubsen J et al (2006) A comparison of the effects of carvedilol and metoprolol on well-being, morbidity, and mortality (the "patient journey") in patients with heart failure: a report from the Carvedilol Or Metoprolol European Trial (COMET). J Am Coll Cardiol 47:1603-1611
38. Conraads VM, Metra M, Kamp O et al (2012) Effects of the long-term administration of nebivolol on the clinical symptoms, exercise capacity, and left ventricular function of patients with diastolic dysfunction: results of the ELANDD study. Eur J Heart Fail 14:219-225
39. Ekman I, Chassany O, Komajda M et al (2011) Heart rate reduction with ivabradine and health related quality of life in patients with chronic heart failure: results from the SHIFT study. Eur Heart J 32:2395–2404
40. Dobre D, van Jaarsveld CH, deJongste MJ et al (2007) The effect of beta-blocker therapy on quality of life in heart failure patients: a systematic review and meta-analysis. Pharmacoepidemiol Drug Saf 16:152-159

41. Volterrani M, Cice G, Caminiti G et al (2011) Effect of carvedilol, ivabradine or their combination on exercise capacity in patients with heart failure (the CARVIVA HF trial). Int J Cardiol 151:218-224
42. Kasper EK, Gerstenblith G, Hefter G et al (2002) A randomized trial of the efficacy of multidisciplinary care in heart failure outpatients at high risk of hospital readmission. J Am Coll Cardiol 39:471-480
43. Jankowska EA, Rozentryt P, Witkowska A et al (2010) Iron deficiency: an ominous sign in patients with systolic chronic heart failure. Eur Heart J 31:1872-1880
44. Anker SD, Comin Colet J, Filippatos G et al (2009) Ferric carboxymaltose in patients with heart failure and iron deficiency. N Engl J Med 361:2436-2448
45. Belardinelli R, Georgiou D, Cianci G et al (1999) Randomized, controlled trial of long-term moderate exercise training in chronic heart failure. Effects on functional capacity, quality of life and clinical outcome. Circulation 99:1173-1182
46. Tyni-Lenne R, Gordon A, Jensen-Urstad M et al (1999) Aerobic training involving a minor muscle mass shows greater efficacy than training involving a major muscle mass in chronic heart failure patients. J Cardiac Fail 5:300-307
47. Willenheimer R, Erhardt L, Cline C et al (1998) Exercise training in heart failure improves quality of life and exercise capacity. Eur Heart J 19:774-781
48. Klocek M, Kubinyi A, Bacior B et al (2005) Effect of physical training on quality of life and oxygen consumption in patients with congestive heart failure. Intern J Cardiol 103:323-329
49. Sledge SB, Ragsdale K, Tabb J et al (2000) Comparison of intensive outpatient cardiac rehabilitation to standard outpatient care in veterans: effects on quality of life. J Cardiopulmon Rehabil 20:383-388
50. Owen A, Croucher L (2000) Effect of an exercise programme for elderly patients with heart failure. Eur J Heart Fail 2:65-70

Quality of Life in Patients with Cardiac Rhythm Disturbances

6

Bogumiła Bacior and Katarzyna Styczkiewicz

6.1 Introduction

In recent years, radical changes have been observed in the treatment of disturbances in cardiac rhythm. Multicenter clinical studies have allowed for better understanding of the pathogenesis of rhythm disturbances. Treatment options have been aimed at reducing mortality and improving health-related quality of life (HRQoL). Despite advances in pharmacotherapy and electrotherapy, many patients with rhythm disturbances experience various symptoms which often do not allow them to participate in everyday activities. Though the circumstances surrounding the occurrence of arrhythmia are unpredictable, the QoL of patients is influenced by the frequency and duration of attacks as well as the degree to which symptoms are exacerbated. Sudden and frequent hospitalizations due to arrhythmia as well as the side effects of antiarrhythmic drugs also constitute a severe burden for patients.

6.2 Influence of Atrial Fibrillation (AF) on HRQoL

AF is the most frequent atrial tachyarrhythmia and the third most often encountered arrhythmia. It is also the leading cause of hospitalization due to rhythm disturbance. The number of people hospitalized due to AF continues to increase. This trend is the result of an aging population and an increased incidence of congestive heart failure. AF is a common problem in subjects with hypertension, especially in those with concomitant left ventricular hypertrophy. Hypertension increases the risk of AF by up to fourfold.

B. Bacior (✉)
I Department of Cardiology and Hypertension
Jagiellonian University Medical College, Kraków, Poland
e-mail: bacior@cm-uj.krakow.pl

K. Kawecka-Jaszcz et al. (eds.), *Health-Related Quality of Life in Cardiovascular Patients*,
DOI: 10.1007/978-88-470-2769-5_6 © Springer-Verlag Italia 2013

The natural history of AF begins from short attacks which are often asymptomatic. Frequently immune to intervention, these attacks gradually grow into ever longer arrhythmic episodes, resulting in permanent AF, which is classified as "newly diagnosed AF" or "recurrent AF". Recurrent AF describes three types of arrhythmia based on the length of the incident and mechanism for returning to sinus rhythm: paroxysmal, persistent, and permanent [1]. Each type of AF leads to various symptoms, including palpitations, dizziness, intolerance to physical activity, fatigue, chest pain, dyspnea, and syncope. All yield a significantly negative influence on HRQoL.

Initially, the goal of all pharmacologic and invasive interventions for AF was to decrease mortality and the incidence of complications, while effectively controlling cardiac rhythm. However, little attention was devoted to HRQoL [1]. As a result, a continuously growing interest in HRQoL has generated various studies in AF patients.

6.3 Assessing HRQoL in Subjects with AF

Most studies examining QoL concentrate on four main domains: physical fitness, psychological state, social functioning, and everyday functioning [2, 3]. The following are the most of used questionnaires to measure HRQoL in AF patients: Medical Outcomes Study Short Form Health Survey 36 (SF-36) [4], Symptom Checklist (SCL) [5], Atrial Fibrillation Severity Scale [6], Specific Symptom Scale [6], Specific Activity Scale [7], Quality of Life Index-Cardiac Version III [8], Minnesota Living with Heart Failure [9], Quality of Wellbeing Scale [10], Psychological General Wellbeing Index [11], Karolinska Questionnaire (KQ) [12], and the Pacemaker Symptom Scale (PSS) [13].

At present, SF-36 is the most recognized and accepted standardized questionnaire used to measure general QoL in AF patients [1, 4]. The questionnaire consists of eight scales that measure: physical fitness; pain; restrictions placed on activities resulting from physical or emotional reasons; social activity; degree of life activity; mental health; and self-rated general health. Each scale is represented as a value from 0 to 100, whereby a low score reflects low HRQoL.

SCL and KQ are two well-developed, detailed questionnaires used to measure (among others) HRQoL in AF patients [5, 12]. The results are summed for the incidence of complaints and their exacerbation. All the other questionnaires present results separately for each type of symptom, which makes subsequent interpretation of these results difficult but helps to define the symptom which is most improved after a given intervention. Other often encountered questionnaires include the Specific Symptom Scale (used in subjects with AF and congestive heart failure) [7], and PSS (used to assess symptoms in patients with implantable pacemakers) [13].

Widespread use of SF-36 and the other questionnaires mentioned above allows comparison between many studies, but the scales may not be sufficiently sensitive to be used to detect disease-specific changes in HRQoL. Recently, several studies concentrated on development of AF-specific and more comprehensive HRQoL questionnaires. There have been attempts to develop the protocols in Japanese and Spanish populations [14, 15]. Of note is a newly developed and validated HRQoL questionnaire by Spertus et al. [16]. The 20-item Atrial Fibrillation Effect on Quality-of-life (AFEQT) questionnaire provides a 4-item symptoms score, an 8-item daily activities score, a 6-item treatment concerns score, and a 2-item treatment satisfaction scale from which individual domain and global scores are calculated. This questionnaire, in contrast to generic HRQoL tools, contains questions pertaining exclusively to issues relevant to AF patients, and therefore may be more sensitive to subtle changes in HRQoL.

6.4 AF and HRQoL: Descriptive Studies

The importance of distinguishing between subjects with asymptomatic AF and healthy individuals was underlined by Saveliev et al. who, when using SCL to measure the incidence and severity of symptoms, did not find significant differences in HRQoL between these two groups [17]. However, when using SF-36, asymptomatic AF patients were characterized by lower scores of global life-satisfaction and lower self-rated health. Compared with asymptomatic patients and healthy individuals, symptomatic AF patients had a significantly lower HRQoL score in all domains of the SF-36. This means that the greater the incidence and severity of AF symptoms, the greater the negative influence on HRQoL.

There have been several studies focusing on the measurement of HRQoL in patients with paroxysmal and permanent AF [18, 19]. Dorian et al. noted that 90% of patients with paroxysmal or permanent AF presented with symptoms of palpitations, dyspnea, and limited exercise performance [18]. Surprisingly, patients with paroxysmal AF had a lower HRQoL across all domains of the SF-36, similar to that seen in patients after myocardial infarction. The paroxysmal AF patients were affected by symptoms associated with attacks of AF, limited exercise performance, and symptom severity. The authors speculated that measured HRQoL was not dependent upon objective indicators used in medicine to indicate disease severity.

More recent published data were in accordance with this study, and confirmed that patients with uncontrolled symptomatic paroxysmal AF at baseline had lower HRQoL than patients with controlled symptomatic paroxysmal AF [20]. However, treatment with flecainide improved their HRQoL to a level comparable with that seen in control patients.

In another study focusing on subjects with permanent AF, a questionnaire containing open questions found that the incidence of symptoms decreased global HRQoL, and had a negative effect on the everyday functioning of patients [19].

Hagens et al. evaluated patients with paroxysmal AF using SF-36 and found decreased HRQoL in the dimensions of physical, social, and intellectual functioning [21]. Lower HRQoL did not, however, relate to objective health indicators such as left ventricular ejection fraction, New York Heart Association (NYHA) class, or symptoms related to arrhythmia. It was noted that chest pain and weakness (symptoms commonly associated with attacks of AF) significantly influenced HRQoL (i.e., a lower score in terms of physical ability).

It is not known if HRQoL is more influenced by the presence of paroxysmal or permanent AF. Concomitant diseases such as hypertension, coronary artery disease, congestive heart failure, or valvular heart disease often accompany AF. This makes interpretation of questionnaire results much more difficult. HRQoL differences based on sex have also been noted among AF patients. Compared with men, the Canadian Trial of Atrial Fibrillation (CTAF) found that women with AF had lower indicators of physical fitness and more advanced symptoms even after adjusting for age as well as clinical and demographic factors [22].

6.5 Influence of AF Treatment on HRQoL

AF constitutes a significant and frequently encountered problem in everyday clinical practice, but consensus on the optimal treatment of arrhythmia is lacking. Two alternative approaches exist: (i) returning to sinus rhythm or (ii) leaving the arrhythmia while regulating ventricular rhythm and offering anticoagulation therapy. Both strategies, however, have various restrictions. Returning an AF patient to sinus rhythm seems to be a natural goal. It allows physiologic control of cardiac rhythm, improves cardiac output and physical tolerance, and decreases symptom severity. However, pharmacotherapy is usually less effective over time, and the frequency of recurring AF after 6-month observation is as high as 50%. A body of data has also revealed increased mortality trends among patients receiving antiarrhythmic treatment [23]. Long-term use of oral anticoagulants may also increase the risk of bleeding complications.

Choosing an "ideal" form of treatment is difficult, but large, randomized double-blind studies cast a new light on AF treatment. The Atrial Fibrillation Follow-up Investigation of Rhythm Management (AFFIRM) is the largest study comparing treatments that consist of returning the patient to sinus rhythm versus treatment comprising leaving the arrhythmia and controlling only ventricular rhythm. A total of 4,060 AF patients were in this study, with an observation period lasting 3–6 years [1]. QoL was determined with tests used to measure general HRQoL (i.e., Perceived Health (PH), Cantril Ladder of Life (CLL), and SF-36) and tests specific for cardiovascular diseases (i.e., QoL Index Cardiac Version III (QoL-III CV) and SCL). With respect to the measured indicators of QoL, the results showed no differences between the two types of treatment. After 1 year of observation, no differences were found in the HRQoL of AF patients and sinus-rhythm patients. However, at the end of the study, improved HRQoL was noted in both groups of patients.

Studies examining these two treatment options were also undertaken in smaller groups of patients. These included the Strategies of Treatment of Atrial Fibrillation (STAF) [24], Rate Control Versus Electrical Cardioversion (RACE) [25], and Pharmacological Intervention in Atrial Fibrillation (PIAF) studies [26]. Though none of these trials showed significant differences in HRQoL between the two treatment groups, within group improvement in HRQoL was noted. In the rhythm-controlling group, the STAF study observed an increase in five dimensions of the SF-36: physical activity; restrictions in fulfilling everyday roles due to physical reasons; pain; social functioning; and psychological health [24]. However, progress was noted in only two dimensions in the sinus-rhythm group: restrictions in fulfilling everyday roles due to physical and psychological reasons [24]. In the PIAF study, using the same questionnaire, Hohnloser et al. found that the rhythm-controlling group had improved vitality, social and physical functioning, and decreased pain [26]. An improvement was also observed in the sinus-rhythm group with regard to: psychological health; vitality level; social and physical functioning; restrictions in fulfilling everyday roles due to physical reasons; and feeling pain [26]. Conversely, the RACE study confirmed improvement only in the rhythm-controlling group noted across three dimensions of the SF-36: restrictions in fulfilling everyday roles due to physical reasons; psychological health; and social functioning [25]. No significant increase in HRQoL was noted in the sinus-rhythm group [25]. Also, no significant differences in HRQoL were found when comparing the two methods with one another. This analysis found the presence of sinus rhythm, shorter time of AF, and younger age to be factors leading to significant improvement in HRQoL.

One can observe a different situation between subjects with AF and those with congestive heart failure patients [27]. When comparing patients with congestive heart failure with those with sinus rhythm or AF, the former exhibited better physical tolerance (i.e., better results for the Six-minute Walking Test) and improved HRQoL after treatment with beta-blockers. Even when using the same treatment, QoL did not change in AF patients [27].

Beside pharmacotherapy, three basic invasive treatment options exist:

- symptomatic treatment: cardioversion, ablation or modifying the atrioventricular (AV) junction, implanting an atrioverter;
- preventing attacks: permanent stimulation;
- treating the cause: eliminating the arrhythmia trigger or preventing the onset and development of re-entry (e.g., ablation, surgical treatment).

Table 6.1 Selected studies on health-related quality of life in subjects with atrial fibrillation treated surgically by the Maze procedure

Study	Number of patients/ observation period	Questionnaire used	Outcome
Lönnerholm [32]	N = 48, AF patients resistant to pharmacologic treatment/1 year	SF-36	- improvement in all domains of the SF-36 with the exception of pain - greatest improvement noted in the dimensions measuring physical functioning
Jessurun [40]	N = 35, AF patients qualified for mitral-valve replacement/1 year	SF-36 SDQ (questionnaire measuring cardiac symptoms, sleep, cognitive functioning, intellectual health, and social functioning)	- after 3 months, in the Maze group, improvement was noted in the SF-36 dimensions of physical functioning and role restrictions due to physical reasons - after 3 months, in the non-Maze group, improvement was noted in the SF-36 dimensions of self-rated general health, functioning, and vitality - after 12 months, no differences were noted between groups with SF-36 or SDQ

AF, atrial fibrillation; *SF-36*, Short Form Health Survey; *SDQ*, Strengths and Difficulties Questionnaire.

The SF-36 was most often used to measure HRQoL in AF patients undergoing invasive treatment (Tables 6.1–6.3).

6.6 Ablation/Modification of the AV Junction with Pacemaker Implantation

Significant improvement in HRQoL has been documented using general and specific questionnaires for this form of AF therapy [6, 28, 29]. Bubien et al. used four questionnaires to measure HRQoL: SF-36, SCL, Perceived Impact of the Arrhythmia on Activities of Daily Living, and Performance of Activities of Daily Living [6]. Patients who had ablation with subsequent pacemaker implantation noted significant improvement in all dimensions of the SF-36 with the exception of general self-rated health.

Table 6.2 Selected studies on health-related quality of life in subjects with atrial fibrillation treated by radiofrequency ablation

Study	Number of patients/ observation period	Questionnaire used	Outcome
Pappone [33]	N = 1171, 589 patients underwent ablation of pulmonary veins, 582 patients were treated only for controlling rhythm/1 year No controls	SF-36	- HRQoL improved only in the ablation group (i.e., physical and psychological functioning)
Gernstenfeld [34]	N = 41, I: electrophysiologic study without ablation (n = 11); II: ablation with recurring arrhythmia (n = 18); III: effective ablation therapy (n = 12)/6 months	SF-36 Measuring symptoms (general questionnaire)	- Group II: improved HRQoL with reduction in symptoms less than in group III - Group III: significant improvement in HRQoL, reduction in symptoms
Wazni [35]	N = 70, with paroxysmal AF, randomized to pulmonary vein antrum isolation by RF ablation or use of flecainide/ sotalol/6 months	SF-36	- Significantly greater improvement in HRQoL in ablation group than in group treated by pharmacological means
Tondo [36]	N = 105, with paroxysmal and persistent AF (40 patients with LVEF < 40% compared with 65 without) pulmonary vein "vestibule" ablation plus linear ablation in mitral isthmus and cavotricuspid isthmus/6 months	SF-36	- Improvement in ≥ 6 measures of SF-36 after ablation - Improvements similar whether or not LV dysfunction present
Wokhlu [37]	N = 323, undergoing RF ablation of AF/2years	SF-36 Mayo Atrial Fibrillation-Specific Symptom Inventory	HRQoL improvement in patients with and without recurrence - AF-specific symptom assessment more accurately reflected ablation efficacy - higher HRQoL when antiarrhythmic drugs were not required after ablation compared with AF controlled with drugs after the procedure

AF, atrial fibrillation; *HRQoL*, health-related quality of life; *RF*, radiofrequency; *SF-36*, Short Form Health Survey.

Table 6.3 Selected studies on health-related quality of life in subjects with atrial fibrillation treated by ablation/modification of the atrioventricular junction with pacemaker implantation

Study	Number of patients/ observation period	Questionnaire used	Outcome
Bubien [6]	N = 161, with supraventricular or ventricular arrhythmia, including 22 with AF/6 months No controls	SF-36 Symptom Checklist - Frequency and Severity; Perceived Impact of the Arrhythmia on Activities of Daily Living; Performance of Activities of Daily Living	- AF patients, compared with those with other arrhythmias, had lower HRQoL - Significant improvement in HRQoL observed after ablation and pacemaker implantation
Ablate and Pace Trial (APT) [28]	N = 156, patients with symptomatic AF, resistant to pharmacotherapy/1 year No controls	Health Status Questionnaire Quality of Life Index, Version III Symptom Checklist: Frequency and Severity	- HRQoL improved across all questionnaires after treatment
Brignole [30]	N = 60, CHF and AF patients, randomized into ablation of the AV junction with implantation of a cardiostimulator or antiarrhythmic pharmacotherapy/1 year	Minnesota Living With Heart Failure Questionnaire (MLHF) Specific Symptoms Scale	- HRQoL improved more with ablation and pacemaker implantation than with pharmacotherapy alone, measured using the symptom questionnaire - No improvement in HRQoL was noted in terms of the MLHF questionnaire

AF, atrial fibrillation; *AV*, atrioventricular; *CHF*, congestive heart failure; *HRQoL*, health-related quality of life; *SF-36*, Short Form Health Survey.

A meta-analysis containing 21 studies and involving 1,181 patients with drug-refractory AF examined the effect of radiofrequency (RF) ablation and pacing therapy on HRQoL. The results demonstrated a significant improvement in HRQoL after the procedure [30].

A systematic review by Thrall et al. suggested that adjunctive pharmacological therapy did not appear to confer additional benefit on HRQoL over ablate and pace procedures alone. The significant improvement in HRQoL demonstrated after ablate and pace procedures may be explained by the marked symptomatic relief such treatment provides [31].

Similar results were found in a study of patients after isolation of pulmonary veins or the Maze procedure. This created an "anatomical barrier" for the conduction and diffusion of arrhythmia [32]. In these patients, besides questions concerning pain, significant improvement was noted in the remaining dimensions of the SF-36, especially with respect to physical and psychological activity.

The Ablate and Pace Trial (APT) noted improvement in HRQoL measured using the Health Status Questionnaire, Quality of Life Index Cardiac Version III, and SCL [28]. Only a select group of patients with difficult-to-control AF attacks participated in this study, so the results could not be generalized for all AF patients. This point is worth remembering if analyzing the results of HRQoL studies comparing patients treated with ablation of the AV junction with pacemaker implantation versus those treated by pharmacological means to control ventricular rhythm.

6.7 RF Ablation

There have been many studies on several techniques that apply RF ablation to treat AF [33–37]. Pappone et al. compared ablation in the area of the pulmonary veins with pharmacological treatment involving control of ventricular rhythm [33]. HRQoL was measured using SF-36 at baseline and every 3 months over 1 year. This study found ablation therapy improved HRQoL whereas antiarrhythmic drugs (i.e., amiodarone, propafenone, sotalol), though effective in controlling ventricular rhythm, did not improve HRQoL.

Using SF-36 and a questionnaire examining symptoms, Gernstenfeld et al. studied 41 patients considered for ablation in the area of the pulmonary veins [34]. Eleven underwent electrophysiologic testing without ablation; 18 had ablation and recurring AF; and 12 had a successful RF ablation.

The greatest improvement in HRQoL was reported by patients after successful ablation, whereas a trend towards improvement, though not as significant, was also noted in patients with recurrent AF after ablation. Other selected available studies are shown in Table 6.2.

A degree of caution is needed when interpreting the HRQoL outcomes available for ablation studies. It appears that some of the symptomatic benefit of ablation is not due to control of the rhythm because investigators have shown an increase in the frequency of asymptomatic AF after ablation [38, 39]. There is also a great potential for placebo and non-placebo effects based on the subjective nature of HRQoL endpoints and the lack of blinding in these studies. It has been shown that invasive cardiac procedures, even under "sham" conditions, can improve patient reported wellbeing [39]. Despite these limitations, catheter ablation for AF appears to be more effective than drugs for rhythm control, and available data suggest that successful procedures are associated with large improvements in HRQoL in highly symptomatic patients.

6.8 Surgical Treatment for AF

The Maze procedure is the best known surgical method of AF treatment [32]. This procedure, because of its invasive character, is sometimes used as an additional procedure, especially in patients with valvular heart disease. Lönnerholm et al. studied patients with lone AF, which constituted 80% of the general sample, as candidates for this procedure [32]. HRQoL was measured using SF-36 before surgery as well as 6 months and 12 months thereafter. The study involved 48 patients who underwent the Maze procedure. Sinus rhythm was restored and maintained in 90% of patients after 6 months of observation. After the procedure, HRQoL improved across all dimensions of the SF-36 with the exception of pain. Six and 12 months after the procedure, HRQoL reached an age-appropriate level characteristic for the general population.

Jessurun et al. studied patients with symptomatic, lone AF resistant to pharmacotherapy treated using the Maze procedure, whereas HRQoL was measured using SF-36 [40]. After this procedure, patients also noted significant improvement in HRQoL.

6.9 HRQoL in Patients with Supraventricular Arrhythmia

Improving QoL is one of the main therapeutic goals in the treatment of supraventricular tachycardia (SVT), atrioventricular nodal reentrant tachycardia (AVNRT), and atrioventricular reentrant tachycardia (AVRT). RF ablation and pharmacotherapy have been proposed as effective treatment strategies. There have been few studies examining to what extent these two strategies differ in their influence on HRQoL.

Previous studies reported that RF ablation improves HRQoL in patients with SVT [6, 41]. Lau et al. examined SVT patients with an additional accessory pathway subject to RF ablation after 3 months of antiarrhythmic therapy [41]. QoL was measured using the General Health Questionnaire, Somatic Symptoms Inventory and Sickness Impact Profile. After RF ablation, improvement in HRQoL was maintained for 1 year of follow-up, and patients observed increased exercise tolerance.

The extent of improvement in HRQoL varied between patients according to the severity of arrhythmia. This observational study was, however, limited to patients with severe symptoms or those who have had undergone previous antiarrhythmic therapy.

A subsequent study [42] compared the influence of RF ablation and pharmacotherapy on the HRQoL of SVT patients. Both strategies improved HRQoL and decreased the frequency of symptoms. However, compared with pharmacotherapy, ablation decreased the frequency of symptoms in more patients (i.e., 74% versus 33%).

In another prospective study, Goldberg et al. [43] compared the long-term influence of RF ablation and pharmacotherapy as initial forms of therapy in 83 patients with newly diagnosed acute SVT (AVNRT 67%; AVRT 28%). HRQoL was measured using SF-36. Improved HRQoL was confirmed in both groups after 1 year. During this time, significant improvement in physical and social functioning was noted in the group receiving pharmacotherapy. However, after 5 years, compared with other baseline measurements, only physical functioning remained significantly improved. In the RF ablation group, at 1 year and 5 years of observation, improvement was noted in physical and emotional dimensions as well as in self-rated psychological health. However, in such dimensions as self-rated general health, bodily pains, social functioning, and vitality, the extent of improvement was lower after 5 years of observation. Compared with their pharmacologically treated counterparts, RF-ablation patients continued to have significantly better indicators of HRQoL even after 5 years of observation. As opposed to those treated using pharmacotherapy, patients treated using ablation reported complete elimination of symptoms (e.g., dizziness, palpitations, syncope) significantly more often (70% versus 43%). Interestingly, at baseline, women had a worse perception of arrhythmia than men. Compared with men, the HRQoL of women was lower across all dimensions of the SF-36. However, after 5 years of observation, in most of the dimensions of the SF-36, women reported greater improvement in QoL than men.

A study by Schaer et al. in a group of 94 patients treated using ablation (62 patients with AVNRT and 32 with AVRT) found that 96% of patients reported arrhythmia symptoms to a lesser extent, expressing a high level of satisfaction after the procedure [44].

In a large retrospective study involving 454 patients undergoing ablation of SVT (AVNRT, AVRT and ectopic atrial tachycardia), HRQoL was assessed at baseline and after 5 years using SF-36 and SCL [45]. Patients treated with RF ablation showed significant reductions in arrhythmia-related symptoms and improvement in physical, emotional and social indices of HRQoL. Only patients with ectopic atrial tachycardia showed a trend towards HRQoL improvement.

Specific paroxysmal symptoms cannot be quantified with general measures of HRQoL such as with SF-36. Hence, there have been attempts made to develop an arrhythmia-specific HRQoL questionnaire for SVT. Of note is a new questionnaire, U22, which measures the: effects of arrhythmia on wellbeing; intensity of discomfort during an episode; type and temporal characteristics of dominant symptoms; duration and frequency of episodes [46]. U22 was used in the evaluation of 88 patients who underwent catheter ablation of SVT, and was found to be useful in quantification of the symptoms associated with SVT.

6.10 HRQoL in Subjects with Vasovagal Syncope

Several studies have found that the prognosis of vasovagal syncope is good and is not associated with an increased risk of sudden cardiac death or increased mortality. However, syncope greatly influences patients' lives, primarily by restricting everyday activities such as driving, operating a machine, or not being able to work [47]. Few data are available on the HRQoL of patients with vasovagal syncope. The 1980s and early 1990s saw some attempts to measure QoL in small groups of such patients. One study examined 62 individuals with recurrent syncope (regardless of cause) using SIP [48]. The results of this study revealed decreased QoL in patients with syncope compared with those with chronic conditions such as rheumatoid arthritis, lower-back pain, or psychiatric diseases.

Rose et al. used the EuroQol-5D (EQ-5D) to evaluate 136 patients with syncope of unknown origin [47]. Compared with the general population, the QoL of syncope patients was lower in all subscales of the EQ-5D: mobility, everyday activities, self-care, pain/discomfort, and anxiety/depression. This study also attempted to measure the relationship between HRQoL and exacerbation of symptoms. A significant negative relationship existed between the frequency of symptoms and HRQoL for patients who experienced ≥ 6 fainting episodes in their lifetime. This was not the case for patients who reported fewer fainting episodes in their medical history. These groups (i.e., < 6 versus > 6 lifetime fainting episodes) had a different prognosis in terms of their risk for recurring syncope: 18% and 50%, respectively [49]. Patients with reduced mobility (measured using EQ-5D) and patients who experienced pain/discomfort resulting from syncope had the lowest HRQoL. Pain/discomfort symptoms most often reflected prodromal symptoms such as dizziness, visual problems, and profuse sweating. Prodromal symptoms decreased HRQoL more than syncope alone.

No therapies have proven useful to improve HRQoL in patients with vasovagal syncope in clinical trials. In the Prevention of Syncope Trial – a randomized, placebo-controlled, double-blind trial – the hypothesis that the beta-blocker metoprolol improves QoL in adult patients with vasovagal syncope in a 1-year observation period was tested [50]. HRQoL was assessed by SF-36 and EQ-5D. The results of the study were negative, and demonstrated that use of metoprolol did not result in improved HRQoL compared with placebo.

References

1. Jenkins LS, Brodsky M, Schron E et al (2005) Quality of life in atrial fibrillation: the Atrial Fibrillation Follow-up Investigation of Rhythm Management (AFFIRM) study. Am Heart J 149:112-120
2. Luderitz B, Jung W (2000) Quality of life in patients with atrial fibrillation. Arch Intern Med 160:1749-1757

3. Gill TM, Feinstein AR (1994) A critical appraisal of the quality of quality-of-life measurements. JAMA 272:619-626
4. Ware JE, Jr, Kosinski M, Bayliss MS et al (1995) Comparison of methods for the scoring and statistical analysis of SF-36 health profile and summary measures: summary of results from the Medical Outcomes Study. Med Care 33 (Suppl 4):S264-279
5. Kang Y, Bahler R (2004) Health-related quality of life in patients newly diagnosed with atrial fibrillation. Eur J Cardiovasc Nurs 3:71-76
6. Bubien RS, Knotts-Dolson SM, Plumb VJ et al (1996) Effect of radiofrequency catheter ablation on health-related quality of life and activities of daily living in patients with recurrent arrhythmias. Circulation 94:1585-1591
7. Brignole M, Gianfranchi L, Menozzi C et al (1994) Influence of atrioventricular junction radiofrequency ablation in patients with chronic atrial fibrillation and flutter on quality of life and cardiac performance. Am J Cardiol 74:242-246
8. Dougherty CM, Dewhurst T, Nichol WP et al (1998) Comparison of three quality of life instruments in stable angina pectoris: Seattle Angina Questionnaire, Short Form Health Survey (SF-36), and Quality of Life Index-Cardiac Version III. J Clin Epidemiol 51:569-575
9. Middel B, Bouma J, de Jongste M et al (2001) Psychometric properties of the Minnesota Living with Heart Failure Questionnaire (MLHF-Q). Clin Rehabil 15:489-500
10. Ganiats TG, Palinkas LA, Kaplan RM (1992) Comparison of Quality of Well-Being scale and Functional Status Index in patients with atrial fibrillation. Med Care 30:958-964
11. Kay GN, Bubien RS, Epstein AE et al (1988) Effect of catheter ablation of the atrioventricular junction on quality of life and exercise tolerance in paroxysmal atrial fibrillation. Am J Cardiol 62:741-744
12. Levy T, Walker S, Rex S et al (2000) Ablate and pace for drug refractory paroxysmal atrial fibrillation. Is ablation necessary? Int J Cardiol 75:187-195
13. Menozzi C, Brignole M, Moracchini PV et al (1990) Intrapatient comparison between chronic VVIR and DDD pacing in patients affected by high degree AV block without heart failure. Pacing Clin Electrophysiol 13:1816-1822
14. Ogawa S, Yamashita T, Yamazaki T (2009) Optimal treatment strategy for patients with paroxysmal atrial fibrillation J-RHYTHM Study. Circulation 73:242-248
15. Arribas F, Ormaetxe JM, Peinado R et al (2010) Validation of the AF-QoL, a disease-specific quality of life questionnaire for patients with atrial fibrillation. Europace 12:364-370
16. Spertus J, Dorian P, Bubien R et al (2011) Development and validation of the Atrial Fibrillation Effect on QualiTy-of-Life (AFEQT) questionnaire in patients with atrial fibrillation. Circ Arrhythm Electrophysiol 4:15-25
17. Savelieva I, Paquette M, Dorian P et al (2001) Quality of life in patients with silent atrial fibrillation. Heart 85:216-217
18. Dorian P, Jung W, Newman D et al (2000) The impairment of health-related quality of life in patients with intermittent atrial fibrillation: implications for the assessment of investigational therapy. J Am Coll Cardiol 36:1303-1309
19. Deaton C, Dunbar SB, Moloney M et al (2003) Patient experiences with atrial fibrillation and treatment with implantable atrial defibrillation therapy. Heart Lung 32:291-299
20. Guédon-Moreau L, Capucci A, Denjoy I (2010) Impact of the control of symptomatic paroxysmal atrial fibrillation on health-related quality of life. Europace 12:634-642
21. Hagens VE, Ranchor AV, Van Sonderen E et al (2004) Effect of rate or rhythm control on quality of life in persistent atrial fibrillation. Results from the Rate Control Versus Electrical Cardioversion (RACE) Study. J Am Coll Cardiol 43:241-247
22. Dorian P, Paquette M, Newman D et al (2002) Quality of life improves with treatment in the Canadian Trial of Atrial Fibrillation. Am Heart J 143:984-990
23. Packer DL, Munger TM, Johnson SB et al (1997) Mechanism of lethal proarrhythmia observed in the Cardiac Arrhythmia Suppression Trial: role of adrenergic modulation of drug binding. Pacing Clin Electrophysiol 20:455-467
24. Carlsson J, Miketic S, Windeler J et al (2003) Randomized trial of rate-control versus rhythm-

control in persistent atrial fibrillation: the Strategies of Treatment of Atrial Fibrillation (STAF) study. J Am Coll Cardiol 41:1690-1696

25. Hagens VE, Crijns HJ, Van Veldhuisen DJ et al (2005) Rate control versus rhythm control for patients with persistent atrial fibrillation with mild to moderate heart failure: results from the RAte Control versus Electrical cardioversion (RACE) study. Am Heart J 149:1106-1111
26. Hohnloser SH, Kuck KH (2001) Randomized trial of rhythm or rate control in atrial fibrillation: the Pharmacological Intervention in Atrial Fibrillation Trial (PIAF). Eur Heart J 22:801-812
27. Fung JW, Chan SK, Yeung LY, Sanderson JE (2002) Is beta-blockade useful in heart failure patients with atrial fibrillation? An analysis of data from two previously completed prospective trials. Eur J Heart Fail 4:489-494
28. Kay GN, Ellenbogen KA, Giudici M et al (1998) The Ablate and Pace Trial: a prospective study of catheter ablation of the AV conduction system and permanent pacemaker implantation for treatment of atrial fibrillation. J Interv Card Electrophysiol 2:121-135
29. Brignole M, Menozzi C, Gianfranchi L et al (1998) Assessment of atrioventricular junction ablation and VVIR pacemaker versus pharmacological treatment in patients with heart failure and chronic atrial fibrillation: a randomized, controlled study. Circulation 98:953-960
30. Wood MA, Brown-Mahoney C, Kay GN et al (2000) Clinical outcomes after ablation and pacing therapy for atrial fibrillation: a meta-analysis. Circulation 101:1138-1144
31. Thrall G, Lane D, Carroll D et al (2006) Quality of life in patients with atrial fibrillation: a systematic review. Am J Med 119:e1-19
32. Lönnerholm S, Blomstrom P, Nilsson L et al (2000) Effects of the maze operation on health-related quality of life in patients with atrial fibrillation. Circulation 101:2607-2611
33. Pappone C, Rosanio S, Augello G et al (2003) Mortality, morbidity, and quality of life after circumferential pulmonary vein ablation for atrial fibrillation: outcomes from a controlled non-randomized long-term study. J Am Coll Cardiol 42:185-197
34. Gerstenfeld EP, Guerra P, Sparks PB et al (2001) Clinical outcome after radiofrequency catheter ablation of focal atrial fibrillation triggers. J Cardiovasc Electrophysiol 12:900-908
35. Wazni OM, Marrouche NF, Martin DO et al (2005) Radiofrequency ablation vs antiarrhythmic drugs as first-line treatment of symptomatic atrial fibrillation: A randomized trial. JAMA 293:2634-2640
36. Tondo C, Mantica M, Russo G et al (2006) Pulmonary vein vestibule ablation for the control of atrial fibrillation in patients with impaired left ventricular function. Pacing Clin Electrophysiol 29:962-970
37. Wokhlu A, Monahan KH, Hodge DO et al (2010) Long-term quality of life after ablation of atrial fibrillation. The impact of recurrence, symptom relief, and placebo effect. JACC 25:2308-2316
38. Lane DA, Lip GYH (2009) Quality of life in older people with atrial fibrillation. J Interv Card Electrophysiol 25:37-42
39. Reynolds MR, Ellis E, Zimetbaum P et al (2008) Quality of Life in Atrial Fibrillation: Measurement Tools and Impact of Interventions. J Cardiovasc Electrophysiol 19:762-768
40. Jessurun ER, van Hemel NM, Defauw JJ et al (2003) A randomized study of combining maze surgery for atrial fibrillation with mitral valve surgery. J Cardiovasc Surg (Torino) 44:9-18
41. Lau CP, Tai YT, Lee PW (1995) The effects of radiofrequency ablation versus medical therapy on the quality-of-life and exercise capacity in patients with accessory pathway-mediated supraventricular tachycardia: a treatment comparison study. Pacing Clin Electrophysiol 18:424-432
42. Bathina MN, Mickelsen S, Brooks C et al (1998) Radiofrequency catheter ablation versus medical therapy for initial treatment of supraventricular tachycardia and its impact on quality of life and healthcare costs. Am J Cardiol 82:589-593
43. Goldberg AS, Bathina MN, Mickelsen S et al (2002) Long-term outcomes on quality-of-life and health care costs in patients with supraventricular tachycardia (radiofrequency catheter ablation versus medical therapy). Am J Cardiol 89:1120-1123

44. Schaer B, Corn TA, Osswald S (2002) Radiofrequency ablation of supraventricular re-entry tachycardia: a "new life" with a successful and complications-free method. Schweiz Rundsch Med Prax 91:216-222
45. Meissner A, Stifoudi I, Weismüller P et al (2009) Sustained high quality of life in a 5-year long term follow-up after successful ablation for supra-ventricular tachycardia. Results from a large retrospective patient cohort. Int J Med Sci 6:28-36
46. Kesek M, Tollefsen T, Glund NH et al (2009) U22, a protocol to quantify symptoms associated with supraventricular tachycardia. PACE 32:S105-S108
47. Rose MS, Koshman ML, Spreng S et al (2000) The relationship between health-related quality of life and frequency of spells in patients with syncope. J Clin Epidemiol 53:1209-1216
48. Linzer M, Pontinen M, Gold DT et al (1991) Impairment of physical and psychosocial function in recurrent syncope. J Clin Epidemiol 44:1037-1043
49. Sheldon R, Rose S, Flanagan P et al (1996) Effect of beta blockers on the time to first syncope recurrence in patients after a positive isoproterenol tilt table test. Am J Cardiol 78:536-539
50. Sheldon RS, Amuah JE, Connolly SJ et al (2009) Effect of metoprolol on quality of life in the Prevention of Syncope trial. J Cardiovasc Electrophysiol 20:1083-1088

Quality of Life in Patients with Implantable Cardiac Devices

7

Bogumiła Bacior, Magdalena Loster and Marek Klocek

7.1 Introduction

In recent years, there has been considerable development in the treatment of arrhythmias and atrioventricular (AV) conduction disturbances through the use of implantable cardiac devices (e.g., pacemakers, cardioverter defibrillators). Such devices may serve several functions, but their primary purpose is to prevent syncope and sudden cardiac death.

7.2 Single- or Dual-Chamber Pacing?

Pacemakers are classified according to the number of cardiac chambers stimulated: one, two, or three. In single-chamber stimulation, the intracardiac lead is located in the right atrium (AAI type of stimulation) or right ventricle (VVI type of stimulation). In dual-chamber stimulation (DDD type of stimulation), two leads are located in the right atrium and right ventricle. These leads preserve AV synchrony, may be more physiological, and can have a rate responsive function that is dependent upon the physical activity of the individual. Three-chamber (i.e., biventricular) stimulation constitutes a relatively new type of electrotherapy in which the third lead is responsible for stimulating the left ventricle.

The health-related quality of life (HRQoL) of subjects with cardio-stimulators is low and comparable with that of the HRQoL of subjects undergoing hemodialysis [1]. However, after implantation, HRQoL improves compared with that observed before the procedure. Gribbin et al. observed improvement in selected areas of

B. Bacior (✉)
I Department of Cardiology and Hypertension
Jagiellonian University Medical College, Kraków, Poland
e-mail: bacior@cm-uj.krakow.pl

K. Kawecka-Jaszcz et al. (eds.), *Health-Related Quality of Life in Cardiovascular Patients*,
DOI: 10.1007/978-88-470-2769-5_7

HRQoL 1 month after the procedure regardless of the type of pacemaker implanted (e.g., VVI, DDD/AAI) [2]. This study used the Schedule for the Evaluation of Individual QoL (SEIQoL) questionnaire, the Short Form Health Survey (SF-36) and the Karolinska Questionnaire (KQ). Both single- and dual-chamber pacing significantly improved SEIQoL scores, cardiovascular symptoms, and the SF-36 domains of mental health, physical and social role limitations.

Młynarski et al. evaluated changes in the primary mental and physical areas of HRQoL in 198 patients 6 months after implantation of a pacemaker because of sinus-node dysfunction or AV block. The Minnesota Living With Heart Failure (MLWHF) questionnaire was used in the study. However, the MLWHF is not designed for patients after pacemaker implantation. A very high statistical improvement in mobility, everyday activity, and pain was found except one: the anxiety/depression dimension in patients with AV block worsened [3].

The question arises as to how different pacing modes influence HRQoL. In terms of hemodynamic advantages such as increasing ejection volume or decreasing pulmonary and right-atrium pressure, short- and long-term clinical studies have demonstrated the superiority of DDD pacemakers over VVI pacemakers. The influence of AV synchrony was then anticipated to include a reduction in critical endpoints and an improvement in QoL. In a study of > 4,500 patients presenting chiefly with sick sinus syndrome (SSS), Lamas, et al. [1] and Connolly, et al. [4] could not prove the advantages of dual-chamber stimulation in terms of overall mortality, cardiovascular mortality, risk of stroke, and the development of atrial fibrillation (AF). Consequently, an attempt was made to measure the greater influence of dual-chamber pacing compared with single-chamber pacing on HRQoL. With this aim, several large, randomized clinical trials were undertaken: the Pacemaker Selection in the Elderly (PASE) study [5], the Canadian Trial of Physiologic Pacing (CTOPP) study [6], and the Mode Selection Trial (MOST) [7].

The aim of the PASE study was to assess HRQoL in 407 patients aged ≥ 65 years who required a permanent pacemaker for the treatment of SSS or AV block [5]. Pacemakers were programmed randomly to ventricular or dual-chamber pacing. HRQoL was assessed using SF-36 and the Specific Activity Scale (SAS) for disease-specific cardiovascular functional status. At the start of the study, according to SF-36, no differences were noted for patients with an indication for pacemaker implantation. After 3 months of follow-up, significant improvement was noted in HRQoL regardless of age, sex, social status, baseline indication for implantation, or previous history of coronary artery disease. QoL improved significantly after pacemaker implantation, but there were no differences between the two pacing modes. No differences were noted between the two forms of stimulation. Also, after 18 months of observation, no differences were noted between ventricular and dual-chamber stimulation in any of the subscales of SF-36. However, after 9-month follow-up, significant differences were noted favoring dual-chamber pacing only in scores for the psychological and emotional health subscale. When measured using the SAS, after 3 months and 9 months of observation, no differences were noted in the HRQoL of either group. However, after 18 months of observation, differences were noted in favor of dual-chamber pacing.

The CTOPP study involved > 2,700 patients randomly divided into "physiologic" (DDD/AAI) or ventricular (VVI) pacing [6]. HRQoL was assessed as a secondary endpoint and measured 6 months after the procedure using the generic scales SF-36, and SAS. As a pacemaker-specific QoL instrument, the Quality of Life Assessment Package (QLAP) was developed on the basis of four domains: physical and psychological health, social functioning, and general activity. The second specific questionnaire used in the study, the Pacemaker Syndrome Scale (PSS), is an instrument measuring "pacemaker syndrome". Pacemaker syndrome refers to symptoms (e.g., dizziness, fatigue) that are potentially attributable to a loss of AV synchrony in patients with ventricular pacing. This study found that VVI and "physiologic" pacing resulted in the same relative magnitude of benefit that was associated with the commencement of pacing. In contrast to the significant effects of receiving a pacemaker, no significant differences in HRQoL could be ascribed to the randomly allocated pacing mode. The authors noted that, in patients with ventricular pacing, pacemaker syndrome was observed less frequently than found in other studies, and that the symptoms of pacemaker syndrome were present less often than in patients with dual-chamber pacing.

The MOST was designed in a similar manner to the CTOPP Trial, in which 2,000 patients with SSS were evaluated after pacemaker implantation programmed for VVI or DDD/AAI pacing [7]. They were then followed up for 2 years, with HRQoL being analyzed using SF-36 and SAS. A comparison of these two groups found no statistical differences in QoL. However, 18.3% of 996 randomly selected patients tolerated ventricular pacing poorly due to AV asynchrony. Symptoms included palpitations, syncope, and dizziness. HRQoL improved across all dimensions after reprogramming to dual-chamber pacing.

Chudzik et al. [8] also offered interesting data from a group of 55 patients with stable AF treated using an implanted pacemaker in which VVI stimulation frequencies of 80 per min and 40 per min were compared. The HRQoL of each participant was measured at baseline and after 7 days of observation using a trial-developed questionnaire. A frequency of 80 per min was found to be more advantageous, allowing not only for improved hemodynamic parameters, but also improved HRQoL by decreasing the symptoms connected with fast and irregular heart rate.

7.3 Pacemakers with Rate-Response Functions

In the 1980s, pacemakers with a rate response function began to be used. These adapted the frequency of cardiac stimulation to the physical activity of the patient. These pacemakers allowed for more physiologic pacing, and their hemodynamic benefits were well documented [9]. Compared with pacemakers without this option, HRQoL improved in patients in VVIR and DDDR pacing groups. Though cross-sectional and involving a small sample group, these studies offered valuable insights [9–12]. Patients with rate-responsive pacemakers had a decreased feeling of illness, less shortness of breath, and fewer palpitations [10]. Lau et al. also confirmed a significantly decreased prevalence in shortness of breath and increased energy for everyday activities [9]. Unfortunately, these studies used only generic questionnaires, and their period of observation was limited to only a few weeks.

New tools are being developed to measure more objectively the HRQoL of patients with cardiac diseases treated using implanted devices. Burns et al. administered the Florida Patient Acceptance Survey (FPAS) to 200 patients with a pacemaker, implantable cardioverter-defibrillator (ICD), or implantable atrioverter-defibrillator (ICD-AT) [13]. The FPAS comprises 15 items with four consistent dimensions: return to function; device-related distress; positive appraisal; and body image concerns. This initial investigation of the FPAS suggests that it may be comparable with other methods of measuring HRQoL in patients with implantable devices. Another instrument administered to patients with pacemakers was the MacNew Heart Disease Health-related Quality of Life (MacNew) questionnaire, which was used in the Pacemaker Patients Quality of Life (PAPQoL) study [14]. The MacNew was comparable with the well-known and standardized SF-36, showing its value in measuring HRQoL in patients with implantable devices (see Appendix).

In summary, one can observe improved QoL in patients after pacemaker implantation. However, dual-chamber pacing has not been demonstrated to be significantly more effective than single-chamber pacing. This issue is expected to be tackled in large-scale trials with long-term observation in which HRQoL is measured using reliable instruments.

7.4 Cardiac Resynchronization Therapy (CRT) and HRQoL

CRT is a relatively new type of electrotherapy. This biventricular stimulation works by returning inter- and intra-ventricular synchrony. In 2002, this method became recognized as an accepted means of electrostimulation and to be a beneficial treatment option for patients with end-stage heart failure. At present, biventricular pacing (BVP) constitutes the most dynamically developed form of cardiac electrostimulation [15].

Studies examining the value of simultaneous biventricular stimulation in cases of congestive heart failure (CHF) have been ongoing for many years. Several multicenter studies have taken place: Multi-Sensor Monitoring in Congestive Heart

Table 7.1 Studies examining health-related quality of life in subjects undergoing cardiac resynchronization therapy

Study (year)	NYHA class	Number of patients	Influence on HRQoL
MUSTIC (2001)	III	67	Significant improvement
PATH-CHF I (2002)	III–IV	42	Significant improvement
PATH-CHF II (2003)	II–IV	101	Significant improvement
MIRACLE (2002)	III–IV	453	Significant improvement
InSync ICD (2002)	II–IV	84	Significant improvement
MIRACLE ICD (2003)	III–IV	369	Significant improvement
CONTAK CD (2003)	II–IV	490	Trend towards improvement, lacking statistical significance; significant improvement only in subgroups of NYHA class III–IV patients
COMPANION (2004)	III–IV	1,520	Significant improvement
CARE-HF (2005)	III–IV	813	Significant improvement

NYHA, New York Heart Association; *HRQoL*, health-related quality of life.

Failure (MUSTIC) [16]; Pacing Therapies for Congestive Heart Failure (PATH-CHF I) [17]; PATH-CHF II [18]; Multicenter InSync Randomized Clinical Evaluation (MIRACLE) [19]; InSync ICD [20]; Multicenter InSync ICD Randomized Clinical Evaluation (MIRACLE ICD) [21]; CONTAK CD [22]; Comparison of Medical Therapy, Pacing and Defibrillation in Heart Failure (COMPANION) [23]; and Cardiac Resynchronization Heart Failure (CARE-HF) [24]. These studies took place among patients with advanced CHF (i.e., classes III and IV according to the New York Heart Association (NYHA) scale), left ventricular dysfunction (i.e., ejection fraction < 35%), and wide QRS waves on electrocardiography. In all patients, symptoms of CHF were present despite optimal pharmacotherapy (i.e., angiotensin-converting enzyme inhibitors, beta-blockers, loop diuretics, spironolactone, digoxin).

These studies confirmed the effectiveness of BVP expressed through improved tolerance and NYHA functional class. In 2003, CRT was first confirmed to reduce mortality in CHF patients (COMPANION study) [25] and, through a meta-analysis of published randomized studies, mortality related to CHF [26].

The studies that also measured HRQoL as a primary or secondary endpoint are given in Table 7.1. MUSTIC was the first study to confirm long-term advantages after the use of CRT. The HRQoL of NYHA class-III patients, be they in AF or sinus rhythm, was measured using two questionnaires: Minnesota Living with Health Failure (MLHF) questionnaire (which was designed specifically for CHF patients) and KQ (used widely among patients with pacemakers). Significant improvement in the measured dimensions of HRQoL was noted after 3 months and 12 months of observation, with a simultaneous decrease in CHF symptoms and better tolerance of physical activity. Improvement was also noted in the HRQoL of AF patients, but not as significantly as in patients in sinus rhythm [16].

The PATH-CHF I study also measured HRQoL using the MLHF questionnaire, with scores ranging from 0 points (best) to 105 points (worst). Prior to implantation of a biventricular pacemaker, patients rated their HRQoL to a mean value of 48.6 points. After implantation, this score dropped to 20 points ($p < 0.001$) [17]. Similar results were obtained in the PATH-CHF II study, which used the same questionnaire to measure QoL in a larger group of patients [18].

In contrast to the studies mentioned above, MIRACLE was the first randomized, prospective study with a double-blind sample involving a larger number of patients. This allowed for a wider measure of HRQoL in CHF patients with CRT, in which significant improvement was noted in QoL using the MLHF questionnaire (25).

The MLHF questionnaire was also used in the prospective InSync ICD study (26). Participants in NYHA classes II–IV had a low baseline HRQoL (mean, 53 points). CRT led to significant improvement in HRQoL after 1 month of treatment (mean, 31 points). This improvement was sustained after 3 (33 points), 6 (31 points), and 12 (31 points) months of observation. Similar to the studies mentioned above, simultaneous improvement was also noted in CHF symptoms.

MIRACLE ICD, a randomized, double-blind study, compared patients who received devices (i.e., with combined CRT and ICD capabilities) and controls (i.e., ICD activated, but CRT off). Similar to other studies, the MLHF questionnaire was used to measure QoL, and improvement was noted in both groups. However, compared with ICD patients, a significantly greater improvement in the MLHF questionnaire was noted in the CRT + ICD group at 6 months [21].

Only the CONTAK CD study did not find differences in the HRQoL of patients undergoing CRT alone versus CRT + ICD versus ICD alone. This study also used the MLHF questionnaire. Patients with symptomatic CHF (i.e., NYHA classes II–IV) were included in this study. After analyses, significant improvement in HRQoL was noted only in symptomatic CHF patients (i.e., NYHA classes III and IV) [22].

The most important trial was the COMPANION study [23]. This study encompassed 1,520 patients who were randomized into one of three groups: CRT, CRT + ICD, or pharmacotherapy alone. Using the MLHF questionnaire, significant improvement in HRQoL was noted in the groups undergoing CRT as opposed to pharmacotherapy alone. CRT improved the HRQoL of patients with significant left ventricular dysfunction and those with advanced CHF symptoms undergoing optimal pharmacotherapy. In the CARE-HF study, HRQoL measured by the MLHF questionnaire as well as EuroQoL-5D (EQ-5D) improved at 90 days [24].

The question is "which factors might be associated with improvement of HRQoL after CRT? Associations with age, sex, heart failure etiology, QRS width, and ejection fraction before CRT implantation were not found [27]. The only factor that predicted improvement after CRT was functional status (evaluated by NYHA classification). That is, patients with more symptoms of advanced heart failure at baseline responded better to CRT [28, 29].

Evidence that CRT does not "automatically" improve the subjective perception of being "healthier" came from randomized studies in which the device was switched off randomly in some patients whereas in others it remained switched on. After the observation period, an improvement in HRQoL was determined among the patients in whom CRT was switched on [30]. Kloch-Badelek et al. observed significant improvement in HRQoL after CRT implementation but only in a group of "responders" (defined as an increase in walking distance in the 6-minute Walk Test > 10% of baseline values). This finding may mean that patients with advanced heart failure perceive improvement in HRQoL after CRT if their physical ability improves [29].

Mechanical dyssynchrony may also have a role in the identification of subjects who may respond better to CRT. However, recent large clinical trials have challenged this concept. The role of CRT in heart-failure patients with narrow QRS (< 120 ms) is evolving. Such a group of patients was randomly assigned to CRT or optimal pharmacological treatment in the RESPOND study to evaluate clinical responses. HRQoL was assessed by the MLHF questionnaire. Six months after implantation, CRT led to an improvement in HRQoL scores and a reduction of NYHA class. However, no differences in total or cardiovascular mortality emerged between two groups [31].

CRT is mostly achieved by BVP, although it can also be provided by left ventricular pacing (LVP). However, the superiority of BVP over LVP remains uncertain. In 2011, Liang undertook a meta-analysis of randomized controlled trials to compare the effects of two modes of CRT in CHF patients. Outcomes included clinical status besides QoL. Five trials fulfilled the criteria for inclusion in the analysis, which involved 574 patients with CHF indicated for CRT. After a mid-term follow-up, pooled analyses demonstrated that LVP resulted in similar improvements in QoL, as well as other factors of clinical status (6-minute walk distance, NYHA class) [32].

7.5 ICD Therapy and HRQoL

A recognized form of ventricular arrhythmia therapy is implantation of an ICD. During the 1990s, several prospective, randomized studies broadened the indications for using ICD in the primary and secondary prevention of arrhythmia: the Antiarrhythmics Versus Implantable Defibrillators (AVID) [33]; the Canadian Implantable

Defibrillator Study (CIDS) [34]; the Multicenter Automatic Defibrillator Implantation Trial II (MADIT II) [35]; and the Multicenter Unsustained Tachycardia Trial (MUSTT) [36]. Studies focusing on the HRQoL of patients with an ICD found that they tolerated the device, but this acceptance was present only after a certain period of acclimatization to the device (≈6 months). During this period, the HRQoL of the patient (social, economic, and psychological aspects) was also lowest [37]. Unease and anxiety associated with the presence of the ICD device is often observed in patients. Should the device get discharged, increased uneasiness, anxiety, and fear of another discharge or death can be encountered. A subgroup of ICD patients experiences psychological difficulties, with the most profound manifestation being post-traumatic stress disorder [38]. Some patients may even remain in bed for extended periods of time [39]. Only one study did not find a difference in HRQoL between patients with an ICD device that discharged and patients without such an experience [40]. Compared with subjects with cardiovascular disease without an ICD device, most studies confirm a decreased HRQoL in patients after even one discharge [37, 39, 41], and this is influenced by several incidents of ICD discharge [42]. Schron et al. found that even one ICD discharge negatively affected psychological and physical health, whereas > 5 discharges significantly decreased HRQoL [43].

More recent studies have tried to identify predictors of risk of adverse psychological outcomes in subjects with an ICD. The evidence for an influence of ICD implantation and discharges on HRQoL is probably more complex than generally assumed. Symptomatic heart failure [44], younger age [45], poor social support [42], diabetes mellitus [46] and a type-D personality (patients who experience a range of negative emotions but who inhibit the expression of these emotions) [46] constitute other factors that have been associated with a risk of poorer HRQoL outcomes.

Sex has also been proposed to be a potentially important risk factor for poor HRQoL [47]. Sex disparities may be attributed to differences: in the way of dealing with stressful situations; in the acceptance of mechanical devices; in pain sensitivity [48]. Based on these findings, it would be rational to expect women to experience more psychological distress after ICD implantation than men. However, recent studies on sex differences in HRQoL have shown mixed findings. In a multicenter study with a 12-month follow-up of 718 patients, differences in HRQoL were observed for only 2 of 8 subscales of SF-36, with women reporting poorer physical functioning and vitality than men [49].

The Canadian Implantable Defibrillator Study (CIDS) found higher HRQoL in patients with an implanted ICD device compared with those receiving the antiarrhythmic drug amiodarone [50]. This study measured HRQoL in 317 patients using the Mental Health Inventory (MHI) and the Nottingham Health Profile (NHP). Self-rated physical and emotional health improved to a large degree in the ICD group, whereas self-rated emotional health remained unchanged and self-rated physical health worsened in the amiodarone group. However, after analyzing ICD patients who reported > 5 discharges in the previous 12 months, no advantages in terms of HRQoL were noted.

7.6 Conclusions

Improvement in the QoL is observed in most patients after implantation of cardiac devices. It refers mainly to subjects treated with single- or double-chamber pacemakers accompanied with a rate-response function and to CRT. Some studies showed that CRT can improve not only HRQoL, but also the prognosis in heart-failure patients. Conversely, those treated with an ICD device who experienced > 5 discharges may have a deterioration in HRQoL. Symptomatic heart failure, younger age, poor social support, diabetes mellitus, and a type-D personality are factors related to the risk of further decreases in HRQoL.

References

1. Lamas GA, Lee KL, Sweeney MO et al (2002) Ventricular pacing or dual-chamber pacing for sinus-node dysfunction. N Engl J Med 346:1854-1862
2. Gribbin GM, Kenny RA, McCue P et al (2004) Individualised quality of life after pacing. Does mode matter? Europace 6:552-560
3. Mlynarski R, Wlodyka A, Kargul W (2009) Changes in the mental and physical components of the quality of life for patients six months after pacemaker implantation. Cardiol J 16:250-253
4. Connolly SJ, Kerr CR, Gent M et al (2000) Effects of physiologic pacing versus ventricular pacing on the risk of stroke and death due to cardiovascular causes. Canadian Trial of Physiologic Pacing Investigators. N Engl J Med 342:1385-1391
5. Lamas GA, Orav EJ, Stambler BS et al (1998) Quality of life and clinical outcomes in elderly patients treated with ventricular pacing as compared with dual-chamber pacing. Pacemaker Selection in the Elderly Investigators. N Engl J Med 338:1097-1104
6. Newman D, Lau C, Tang AS et al (2003) Effect of pacing mode on health-related quality of life in the Canadian Trial of Physiologic Pacing. Am Heart J 145:430-437
7. Link MS, Hellkamp AS, Estes NA et al (2004) High incidence of pacemaker syndrome in patients with sinus node dysfunction treated with ventricular-based pacing in the Mode Selection Trial (MOST). J Am Coll Cardiol 43:2066-2071
8. Chudzik MMM, Zielińska M, Piestrzewicz K, Goch JK, Kargul W (2004) Wpływ stałej elektrostymulacji serca na parametry hemodynamiczne i jakość życia u pacjentów z utrwalonym migotaniem przedsionków. Folia Cardiologica 11:169-176
9. Lau CP, Rushby J, Leigh-Jones M et al (1989) Symptomatology and quality of life in patients with rate responsive pacemakers: a double-blind, randomized, crossover study. Clin Cardiol 12:505-512
10. Lau CP, Tai YT, Lee PW et al (1994) Quality-of-life in DDDR pacing: atrioventricular synchrony or rate adaptation? Pacing Clin Electrophysiol 17:1838-1843
11. Oto MA, Muderrisoglu H, Ozin MB et al (1991) Quality of life in patients with rate responsive pacemakers: a randomized, cross-over study. Pacing Clin Electrophysiol 14:800-806
12. Staniforth AD, Andrews R, Harrison M et al (1998) "Value" of improved treadmill exercise capacity: lessons from a study of rate responsive pacing. Heart 80:383-386

13. Burns JL, Serber ER, Keim S et al (2005) Measuring patient acceptance of implantable cardiac device therapy: initial psychometric investigation of the Florida Patient Acceptance Survey. J Cardiovasc Electrophysiol 16:384-390
14. Hofer S, Anelli-Monti M, Berger T et al (2005) Psychometric properties of an established heart disease specific health-related quality of life questionnaire for pacemaker patients. Qual Life Res 14:1937-1942
15. Kalinchak DM, Schoenfeld MH (2003) Cardiac resynchronization: a brief synopsis part II: implant and followup methodology. J Interv Card Electrophysiol 9:163-166
16. Cazeau S, Leclercq C, Lavergne T et al (2001) Effects of multisite biventricular pacing in patients with heart failure and intraventricular conduction delay. N Engl J Med 344:873-880
17. Auricchio A, Stellbrink C, Sack S et al (2002) Long-term clinical effect of hemodynamically optimized cardiac resynchronization therapy in patients with heart failure and ventricular conduction delay. J Am Coll Cardiol 39:2026-2033
18. Stellbrink C, Auricchio A, Butter C et al (2000) Pacing Therapies in Congestive Heart Failure II study. Am J Cardiol 86:138K-143K
19. Abraham WT (2000) Rationale and design of a randomized clinical trial to assess the safety and efficacy of cardiac resynchronization therapy in patients with advanced heart failure: the Multicenter InSync Randomized Clinical Evaluation (MIRACLE). J Card Fail 6:369-380
20. Gras D, Leclercq C, Tang AS et al (2002) Cardiac resynchronization therapy in advanced heart failure the multicenter InSync clinical study. Eur J Heart Fail 4:311-320
21. Young JB, Abraham WT, Smith AL et al (2003) Combined cardiac resynchronization and implantable cardioversion defibrillation in advanced chronic heart failure: the MIRACLE ICD Trial. JAMA 289:2685-2694
22. Higgins SL, Hummel JD, Niazi IK et al (2003) Cardiac resynchronization therapy for the treatment of heart failure in patients with intraventricular conduction delay and malignant ventricular tachyarrhythmias. J Am Coll Cardiol 42:1454-1459
23. Bristow MR, Saxon LA, Boehmer J et al (2004) Cardiac-resynchronization therapy with or without an implantable defibrillator in advanced chronic heart failure. N Engl J Med 350:2140-2150
24. Cleland JG, Daubert JC, Erdmann E et al (2005) The effect of cardiac resynchronization on morbidity and mortality in heart failure. N Engl J Med 352:1539-1549
25. Salukhe TV, Francis DP, Sutton R (2003) Comparison of medical therapy, pacing and defibrillation in heart failure (COMPANION) trial terminated early; combined biventricular pacemaker-defibrillators reduce all-cause mortality and hospitalization. Int J Cardiol 87:119-120
26. Bradley DJ, Bradley EA, Baughman KL et al (2003) Cardiac resynchronization and death from progressive heart failure: a meta-analysis of randomized controlled trials. JAMA 289:730-740
27. Krahn AD, Snell L, Yee R et al (2002) Biventricular pacing improves quality of life and exercise tolerance in patients with heart failure and intraventricular conduction delay. Can J Cardiol 18:380-387
28. Faran A, Lewicka-Nowak E, Dabrowska-Kugacka A et al (2008) Cardiac resynchronisation therapy in patients with end-stage heart failure--long-term follow-up. Kardiol Pol 66:19-26; discussion 27
29. Kloch-Badełek M, Klocek M, Czarnecka D et al (2012) Impact of cardiac resynchronization therapy on physical ability and quality of life in patients with chronic heart failure. Kardiologia Polska 6: in press
30. Pinter A, Mangat I, Korley V et al (2009) Assessment of resynchronization therapy on functional status and quality of life in patients requiring an implantable defibrillator. Pacing Clin Electrophysiol 32:1509-1519
31. Foley PW, Patel K, Irwin N et al (2011) Cardiac resynchronization therapy in patients with heart failure and a normal QRS duration: the RESPOND study. Heart 97:1041-1047
32. Liang Y, Pan W, Su Y et al (2011) Meta-analysis of randomized controlled trials comparing isolated left ventricular and biventricular pacing in patients with chronic heart failure. Am J Cardiol 108:1160-1165
33. Klein RC, Raitt MH, Wilkoff BL et al (2003) Analysis of implantable cardioverter defibrilla-

tor therapy in the Antiarrhythmics Versus Implantable Defibrillators (AVID) Trial. J Cardiovasc Electrophysiol 14:940-948
34. Bokhari F, Newman D, Greene M et al (2004) Long-term comparison of the implantable cardioverter defibrillator versus amiodarone: eleven-year follow-up of a subset of patients in the Canadian Implantable Defibrillator Study (CIDS). Circulation 110:112-116
35. Singh JP, Hall WJ, McNitt S et al (2005) Factors influencing appropriate firing of the implanted defibrillator for ventricular tachycardia/fibrillation: findings from the Multicenter Automatic Defibrillator Implantation Trial II (MADIT-II). J Am Coll Cardiol 46:1712-1720
36. Gold MR, Nisam S (2000) Primary prevention of sudden cardiac death with implantable cardioverter defibrillators: lessons learned from MADIT and MUSTT. Pacing Clin Electrophysiol 23:1981-1985
37. Carroll DL, Hamilton GA (2005) Quality of life in implanted cardioverter defibrillator recipients: the impact of a device shock. Heart Lung 34:169-178
38. Versteeg H, Theuns DA, Erdman RA et al Posttraumatic stress in implantable cardioverter defibrillator patients: the role of pre-implantation distress and shocks. Int J Cardiol, 2011 146:438-439
39. Sola CL, Bostwick JM (2005) Implantable cardioverter-defibrillators, induced anxiety, and quality of life. Mayo Clin Proc 80:232-237
40. Duru F, Buchi S, Klaghofer R et al (2001) How different from pacemaker patients are recipients of implantable cardioverter-defibrillators with respect to psychosocial adaptation, affective disorders, and quality of life? Heart 85:375-379
41. Sears SE Jr., Conti JB (2003) Understanding implantable cardioverter defibrillator shocks and storms: medical and psychosocial considerations for research and clinical care. Clin Cardiol 26:107-111
42. Wallace RL, Sears SF, Jr., Lewis TS et al (2002) Predictors of quality of life in long-term recipients of implantable cardioverter defibrillators. J Cardiopulm Rehabil 22:278-281
43. Schron EB, Exner DV, Yao Q et al (2002) Quality of life in the antiarrhythmics versus implantable defibrillators trial: impact of therapy and influence of adverse symptoms and defibrillator shocks. Circulation 105:589-594
44. Johansen JB, Pedersen SS, Spindler H et al (2008) Symptomatic heart failure is the most important clinical correlate of impaired quality of life, anxiety, and depression in implantable cardioverter-defibrillator patients: a single-centre, cross-sectional study in 610 patients. Europace 10:545-551
45. Thomas SA, Friedmann E, Gottlieb SS et al (2009) Changes in psychosocial distress in outpatients with heart failure with implantable cardioverter defibrillators. Heart Lung 38:109-120
46. Pedersen SS, den Broek KC, Theuns DA et al (2009) Risk of chronic anxiety in implantable defibrillator patients: a multi center study. Int J Cardiol 147:420-423
47. Vazquez LD, Conti JB, Sears SF (2010) Female-specific education, management, and lifestyle enhancement for implantable cardioverter defibrillator patients: the FEMALE-ICD study. Pacing Clin Electrophysiol 33:1131-1140
48. Brouwers C, van den Broek KC, Denollet J et al (2011) Gender disparities in psychological distress and quality of life among patients with an implantable cardioverter defibrillator. Pacing Clin Electrophysiol 34:798-803
49. Habibovic M, van den Broek KC, Theuns DA et al (2011) Gender disparities in anxiety and quality of life in patients with an implantable cardioverter-defibrillator. Europace 13:1723-1730
50. Irvine J, Dorian P, Baker B et al (2002) Quality of life in the Canadian Implantable Defibrillator Study (CIDS). Am Heart J 144:282-289

Quality of Life After Stroke

8

Marek Klocek

8.1 Introduction

Stroke constitutes a major medical and social problem, and remains a leading cause of death in industrialized societies. The incidence of stroke and mortality varies among countries. Epidemiological data for stroke obtained for Western Europe and the USA indicate a decrease in incidence and case fatality, whereas those for Central and Eastern Europea show unfavorable results. In Poland, stroke constitutes the fourth leading cause of death, affecting ≈60,000 people every year. Despite stabilized mortality trends due to stroke – 25% in the first month and 40% after 12 months – each year ≈36,000 victims of stroke require permanent treatment and rehabilitation in Poland [1]. In the USA, ≈795,000 people experience a new or recurrent stroke each year. The stroke incidence rate is higher for men compared with women at younger ages, but not at older ages, at which time ≈55,000 more women than men have a stroke [2]. Due to an aging society and improved survival, this number is expected to grow in the coming years. The term "stroke" most often refers to a cerebrovascular incident of atherosclerotic origin. In reality, it refers to various medical conditions not necessarily related to atherosclerosis of cerebral vessels (e.g., stroke after atrial fibrillation (AF) or intracerebral hemorrhage), each with its own prognosis, and possibly requiring separate courses of treatment.

The clinical status of stroke patients is usually measured by their degree of neurological impairment. Neurological symptoms tend to worsen in one-third of patients after a period of time after the stroke. These symptoms usually reach their highest level after 3 days and result from the "evolution of stroke". Being diagnosed with hyperglycemia, pneumonia, or epilepsy are indicative of a worsened prognosis

M. Klocek (✉)
I Department of Cardiology and Hypertension
Jagiellonian University Medical College, Kraków, Poland
e-mail: marek.klocek@wp.pl

K. Kawecka-Jaszcz et al. (eds.), *Health-Related Quality of Life in Cardiovascular Patients*,
DOI: 10.1007/978-88-470-2769-5_8 © Springer-Verlag Italia 2013

during the acute phase. However, measuring the full consequences of stroke should also incorporate: cognitive and intellectual deficits; emotional disturbances; and restrictions in family contacts and social functioning. Cognitive deficits and emotional disturbances negatively influence the time and degree of recovery after stroke.

The effects of stroke include neurological deficits (especially hemiparesis, dysphasia, dysphagia, and cognitive dysfunction) and remit spontaneously in only a small percentage of patients. The vast majority, however, are left handicapped, thereby partially or completely losing independence in everyday activities. The consequences of stroke also include dementia and the need for long-term care, which also tends to affect the caregiver, most often a member of the patient's immediate family [3].

The aim of prevention of primary stroke is to decrease the risk of stroke by reducing the incidence and development of risk factors as well as treating illnesses which may lead to acute cerebrovascular incidents. The most important element of prevention of primary stroke involves the use of oral anticoagulants in patients with AF, effective treatment of hypertension, and treatment of asymptomatic (yet significant) carotid artery stenosis. Hypertension remains the main risk factor for ischemic and hemorrhagic strokes. Its treatment is highly effective in reducing the risk incidence of first-in-a-lifetime stroke. Secondary prevention after a cerebrovascular incident is aimed at preventing recurring stroke, for which there is an ≈10% risk in the first year and a 5–8% risk for each following year. Thus, this risk is estimated to be 30–40% for the first 5 years after the initial stroke, in which time 15% of patients may also suffer a myocardial infarction (MI), with cardiovascular mortality being reported for another 15% of patients [1]. Recurring strokes are associated with a significantly increased risk of death, disability, and healthcare expenses. Risk factors associated with recurring stroke have yet to be defined fully, but are closely related to risk factors associated with the first incident. Transient ischemic attacks (TIAs), characterized by the resolution of acute ischemic symptoms within 24 h, are an important factor predicting stroke. Yet, within 3 months after the first TIA, 10–20% of patients suffer a stroke. As has been shown, one-quarter of all strokes occur in hypertensive patients, whereas the remainder affect normotensive individuals.

Imaging of the central nervous system (CNS) using magnetic resonance imaging (MRI) or computed tomography (CT) can establish the etiology of stroke. However, in many patients, ascertaining precisely the cause of stroke is not possible due to diagnostic difficulties. Some individuals may be asymptomatic, so the incidence of minor stroke in the general population is probably greater than that presented by epidemiologic data. In the absence of neurological complaints in their medical history, CT may show that post-stroke changes have occurred in ≈30% of symptomatic TIA patients and ≈10% of those presenting with acute stroke. The natural history of asymptomatic stroke is not known, though it may be meaningful in the development of vascular dementia. In men and women, the risk for each type of stroke increases exponentially with age. Moreover, patients with symptomatic vascular disease frequently have atherosclerotic changes in the small vasculature in the brain, which are characterized by white matter lesions (WMLs) on MRI [4]. WMLs are often asymptomatic, but they have been indentified as risk factors for functional decline, depression, cognitive impairament and poorer health-related quality of life (HRQoL), mainly due to a developing decline in mental functioning [4]. The prevalence of stroke is ≈30% greater in men than in women, with this difference being most pronounced between 45 years and 65 years of age, and disappearing in older age. Modifiable risk factors for stroke include hypertension, smoking, a high sodium diet, and alcohol abuse.

8.2 HRQoL in Post-Stroke Patients

Suffering a stroke produces many, often dramatic and irreversible, effects in the lives of patients. Stroke may have a remarkably varied effects on how HRQoL is perceived by the patient. While "objectively" analyzing the situation of post-stroke patients, one may expect a decrease in HRQoL, which is confirmed by a significant number of post-stroke patients who rate their HRQoL as very poor or even "worse than death". However, other patients, especially those noting improvement in the initial neurological deficits, begin to report exceptionally high HRQoL. This phenomenon, is called the "disability paradox" or "response shift". Finally, unlike other cardiovascular diseases (CVDs), nowhere is such wide variation in HRQoL scores noted between patients, physicians, and immediate family, as there is in stroke [5].

Varying levels of paralysis-related restrictions in physical activity may constitute a problem for post-stroke patients. CNS damage may also lead to: dysphasia; cognitive and intellectual disturbances; restricted consciousness: and emotional and self-identity disturbances. Compared with restrictions in physical activity, deficits in psychosocial functioning often appear to cause greater problems in post-stroke patients [6]. Conversely, stroke causes a significant decrease in QoL also among those who do not have a post-stroke disability [7].

How HRQoL is measured in post-stroke patients is influenced greatly by the time duration after the stroke (e.g., directly or a few years after). Many longitudinal studies have been limited by short follow-up and enrollment of patients in different stages of early post-stroke recovery. Therefore, measuring HRQoL in post-stroke patients is an important addition to conventional evaluations of health status, in which attention is focused mainly on neurological deficits. Individuals 15–20 years after stroke represent < 10% of all cases but report relatively high HRQoL [8]. For

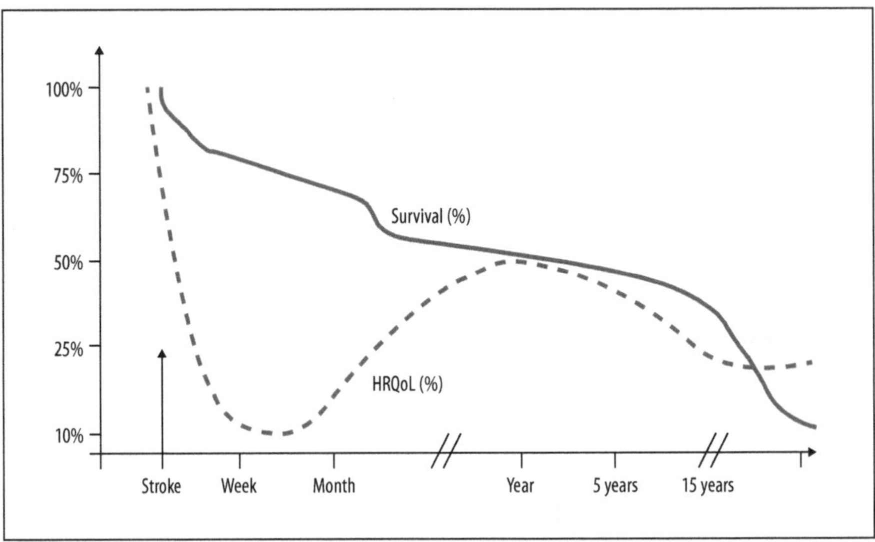

Fig. 8.1 Survival and health-related quality of life in post-stroke patients (100% represents the highest level of health-related quality of life)

example, individuals with 6-year post-stroke survival represented ≈50% of participants in the Auckland Stroke Study but reported relatively high HRQoL [9]. This was the case despite gradually progressing physical disability and increasing dependence on others. In this study, post-stroke HRQoL in women was significantly lower than that for age-matched men, a result found in other illnesses. The schematic relationship between survival and post-stroke HRQoL is presented in Figure 8.1.

HRQoL directly after stroke is low and is dependent upon the severity of neurological deficits (Fig. 8.1). The health state utility of patients after a moderately severe stroke has been found to be one-third that encountered in good health, and is significantly worse than in subjects on dialysis or those who have congestive heart failure (Table 8.1). Though the HRQoL of patients gradually improves after the acute phase of stroke, assuming there is not a complete recovery from neurological deficits, it usually never returns to the same state as before the cerebrovascular incident. Most patients continue to experience different types of restrictions. Hence, the maximum attainable post-stroke HRQoL, after appropriate treatment and rehabilitation, can reach only moderate values. In addition, depression and resignation from social roles (e.g., professional activity) are often the complications of stroke. A high risk of death after stroke has also been observed, which means that improvement in HRQoL concerns only a small percentage of patients under long-term observation.

Table 8.1 Comparison of the health status utility and health-related quality of life for selected health situations or conditions (based on selected data from [10] and [11])

Health status	Health state utility	Health-related quality of life
Good health, no dysfunctions	1.00	Very good
Side effects of hypertension treatment	0.95–0.98	
Mild angina pectoris	0.90	Good
Hypertension and diabetes mellitus	0.86	
Moderate angina and post-mild myocardial infarction	0.70	
Recurring strong pain leading to restrictions of role and professional activity	0.67	Moderate
Dialysis	0.5–0.6	
Mild stroke and transient ischemic attack	0.5–0.7	
Severe angina pectoris, symptomatic congestive heart failure	0,50	
Chronic anxiety, depression, or chronic isolation	0.45	
Need for long-term hospitalization	0.33	Low
Mobility dependent on using mechanical devices	0.31	
Significant and chronic difficulties with memory, orientation, and ability to learn	0.31	
Moderately severe stroke with hemiparesis	0.25–0.30	
Severe stroke with hemiparesis	0.01–0.25	
Death (reference value)	0.00	0
Bilateral paralysis, blindness, severe depression	< 0.00	Unknown
Bedridden due to severe pain and being fully dependent upon others	< 0.00	Unknown
Long-term unconsciousness	< 0.00	Unknown

8.3 Measuring Post-Stroke HRQoL and its Determinants

Measuring HRQoL in post-stroke patients is complex [12]. It is influenced by: conceptual difficulties; variability in the dimensions used to examine HRQoL; different degrees of disease advancement; and the necessity to incorporate the individual needs and preferences of the patient. Hence, measuring improvement in the HRQoL of post-stroke patients requires a complex analysis [13]. Studies undertaken in recent years confirm the view that measuring the neurological state and disability of post-stroke patients does not sufficiently reflect their general functional status. Conversely, measuring HRQoL can offer a more comprehensive view of the patient's current state.

Questionnaires measuring HRQoL after stroke are used mainly to reach two goals. The first goal is to classify patients according to their current psychological and physical abilities or prognosis. For example, when planning to evaluate the effectiveness of a post-stroke rehabilitation program, one may exclude patients with minimal damage to the CNS and those with severe damage to the CNS such that neither group would note significant improvement through rehabilitation. The second goal is to achieve a multidimensional measurement of change through treatment or rehabilitation in the health status and wellbeing of patients.

Though many questionnaires are available to measure HRQoL in stroke patients, only a few can be recommended for widespread use. This is due to a lack of reliable studies concerning the psychometric properties of certain questionnaires. The most often used general questionnaires are the Sickness Impact Profile (SIP), Short Form Health Survey (SF-36), and Nottingham Health Profile (NHP). Other questionnaires used in post-stroke patients include: Karnofsky Performance Status Scale (KPSS); London Handicap Scale; Stroke Adapted Sickness Impact Profile (SA-SIP30); EuroQoL-5D (EQ-5D); Short Form Health Survey 12 (SF-12); Stroke Impact Scale (SIS); McMasters Health Index Questionnaire; Quality of Life Index (QLI); Schedule for the Evaluation of Individual Quality of Life-Direct Weight (SEIQoL-DW); Quality of Wellbeing Scale (PGWB); Newcastle Stroke-Specific Quality of Life Measure (NEWSQOL); Burden of Stroke Scale (BOSS); and the Stroke Specific Quality of Life Scale (SS-HRQoL Scale) (see Appendix).

KPSS was one of the earliest instruments used to measure the functional status and physical activity of patients with chronic diseases (including stroke). At present, it is seldom used. This instrument measures the ability of subjects to work and look after themselves. It also gauges the need for different types of assistance, including the need for hospitalization. One should not forget about detailed scales that allow measurement of specific functional dimensions. For example, the Mini Mental State Examination (MMSE) is used to measure cognitive functioning; the Barthel Index (BI) and the Modified Rankin Scale (MRS) measure disability; and depression can be assessed using the Beck Depression Scale or the Zung Depression Scale (see Appendix). Disability scales (e.g., BI or MRS) correlate poorly with the psychosocial status of patients. Hence, they cannot be used as the only measurements of HRQoL. However, they are used to determine the relationship between an observed level of disability and HRQoL dimensions related to physical health. For example, it has been found that the BI, which measures independent functioning on a scale from 0 (i.e., full dependence) to 20 (i.e., full independence), and the MRS correlate well with the results of the Health Utilities Index (HUI) questionnaires versions 2 and 3, as well as the EQ-5D Index. There are also depression scales which correlate well with the second part of the EQ-5D questionnaire (i.e., EQ-VAS) [14].

Attention has recently been drawn to the fact that certain post-stroke patients cannot rate their HRQoL as a result of severe neurological deficits. Hence, questionnaires using utility measures completed by spouses or caregivers should be used. The results obtained reflect adequately the HRQoL of this group of patients.

8.4 Depression in Post-Stroke Patients

Depression, physical disability, and aggravated cognitive deficits resulting from damaged gray matter and white matter are the main clinical factors influencing decreased HRQoL in stroke patients. Other factors that affect worsening QoL include: difficulty in being understood; poor memory; secondary personality disorders; decreased intellectual functioning; and difficulty in controlling and expressing emotion (e.g., apathy, depressed mood).

Within the first year after stroke, the prevalence of depression in patients with hemiparesis is estimated to be 25–50% [15]. Already in the acute phase, during hospitalization, depression affects ≈20% of patients with stroke. This percentage increases with time. A review by Hackett et al. [16] of studies examining the relationship between stroke and depression estimated its prevalence to be ≈33%. Depression after a cerebrovascular incident does not remain in a direct relationship with the exacerbation of neurological deficits. However, depression tends to occur most often in patients affected by a stroke in the frontal areas of the left hemisphere [17] and in some subcortical areas [18]. Despite relatively minor motor deficits, depression after stroke may inhibit or not permit rehabilitation. Post-stroke depression is therefore a strong determinant of HRQoL in patients, and also influences their long-term prognosis [18].

8.5 Cognitive Function in Post-Stroke Patients

When discussing the HRQoL of stroke patients, special attention should be paid to the development of cognitive dysfunction. This is due to its direct influence on HRQoL as well as difficulties connected with completing the self-assessment type of questionnaires. However, questionnaires have recently been developed which should remedy this problem [19]. Cognitive dysfunction and difficulties connected with independently completing questionnaires occur regardless of the location of the stroke. For example, a left sided stroke usually causes dysphasia as well as difficulty with reading and writing. Conversely, the result of a right-sided stroke may be anosognosia (i.e., denying one's new physical restrictions and functional handicaps). This is sometimes called "hidden dysfunction" which, at cursory examination, may be overlooked by patients and physicians even though it occurs in a significant number of patients [20]. It is characterized by: rapid exhaustion following intellectual activity (e.g., concentration and memory); susceptibility to irritation; mood swings; decreased tolerance for stress; and sensitivity to sound and light ("astheno-emotional syndrome").

8.6 Determinants of Change in the HRQoL of Patients After Stroke

The North East Melbourne Stroke Incidence Study (NEMESIS) study [21] found that, 2 years post-stroke, ≈50% of patients rated their HRQoL as "low" and 25% rated it as "very low" (i.e., < 10% of the HRQoL of healthy individuals). Other studies found that, 6 months post-stroke, physical and psychosocial functioning were the most negatively affected HRQoL dimensions, whereas "treating life as a value" was one of the least affected dimensions. Despite a decrease in HRQoL in the dimension of physical functioning, the authors of these studies reported that patients preserved a positive HRQoL in the dimensions of life satisfaction and family situation. Interestingly, despite definite restrictions in functioning, the level of life satisfaction of stroke patients may be relatively high even after a few months after the incident.

Self-rated HRQoL is dependent upon one's current neurological state and the ability to care for one's self, i.e., functional independence. It seems that rehabilitation geared towards increasing the independence of stroke patients, decreasing isolation, treating depression, and strengthening social support may contribute to improving the HRQoL of stroke patients.

In the early stages after stroke, the HRQoL of patients is determined by various demographic and clinical factors, including age, sex, level of social support, quality of medical care, severity of stroke, depression, and concomitant diseases [22, 23]. Degree of independence in everyday functioning is one of the most important factors influencing HRQoL. For example, van Exel et al. [24] confirmed that the HRQoL of stroke patients is strongly associated with their degree of independence in everyday activities.

In this study, stroke patients, who regained complete independence 2 months and 6 months after the incident, rated their HRQoL (using EQ-5D) at levels similar to the HRQoL of age-matched individuals who had not suffered a stroke (i.e., ≈75% of maximum HRQoL). However, in stroke patients significantly or completely dependent upon external care, HRQoL was very low (i.e., from –14% to +10% of maximum HRQoL).

One method for improving the independence of stroke patients is physical rehabilitation. This focuses especially on paralyzed upper limbs, which supports long-term improvement in HRQoL even after stopping rehabilitation exercises.

A study measuring changes in HRQoL using SF-36 occurring between the fourth and sixteenth month post-stroke in a group of 304 patients [25] found improvement after 1 year in terms of the socioeconomic and psychological dimensions of HRQoL and deteriorating values for physical functioning. Improvement in HRQoL was greater for men, younger patients, and those without symptoms of depression. The psychophysical state of patients significantly influenced the HRQoL of their informal caregivers, whose HRQoL was found to be equally as low in the emotional and psychological dimensions of SF-36 as in patients [25]. This observation, as suggested above, further shows the burden that caring for a stroke patient may have on family functioning [26]. This study also confirmed the chronic influence of depression on the HRQoL of stroke patients.

The NEMESIS study [27] recently published their results involving almost 1,000 patients; 5-year survival was noted in 45%. The vast majority of patients rated their HRQoL as "poor", and 20% as "very poor". Old age, low socioeconomic status, and deepening neurological deficits were predictors of poor HRQoL 5 years after stroke. It was also shown in other studies that the risk of death due to stroke was highest in the lowest-income group in men and women.

A study by Kase et al. [28] involving participants from the Framingham program found that the cognitive functioning of stroke patients (measured using MMSE) was disrupted before the incident. It was therefore subject to significantly greater deterioration, especially in the case of patients with widespread, left-sided stroke. A similar relationship was observed on numerous occasions if decreased HRQoL acted as an early predictor for first stroke [29, 30]. In this study, which looked at the last 13 years of patients' lives, a gradual decline in intellectual functioning took place independently of concomitant depression, leading researchers to suggest that two processes were involved.

Other factors leading to a greater decline in cognitive functioning in stroke patients include untreated or inadequately controlled hypertension that is present before the incident. Hypertension leads to chronic, subclinical brain damage, resulting in a decreased ability to adapt in cases of stroke.

Another observation from the Framingham study concerns dementia after stroke [6]. Having a stroke doubles the risk of developing dementia, regardless of location and severity, sex, age, and concomitant risk factors (e.g., hypertension, AF, diabetes mellitus (DM), smoking). In this study, post-stroke dementia developed in 19.3% of patients, with the risk of development being higher in younger patients with a higher level of education. In the pharmacotherapy of post-stroke dementia, donepezil (a reversible inhibitor of acetylocholine esterase) positively influences the HRQoL of patients [31].

Stroke mostly affects individuals in advanced age, and is the main cause of disability in this group. In the acute phase of stroke, patients may require mechanical ventilation. Measured after 6 months, it has been found that such a course leads to definite improvement in the functional state and HRQoL (i.e., better self-rated physical health, measured using SF-36) of patients. However, this is the case in only one-quarter of patients of advanced age who survive the acute phase.

After stroke, patients often complain about chronic fatigue ("post-stroke fatigue" (PoSF)). This complaint is associated with: a less good prognosis for neurological improvement; worse long-term functioning; definitive decreases in HRQoL; increased mortality [32, 33]. The etiology of PoSF is incompletely understood and its long-term influence on the everyday functioning of stroke patients requires further study [34]. PoSF is present in the acute phase and may affect twice as many patients as post-stroke depression [32].

Pain is another often-encountered symptom after stroke. A high percentage of patients (38–80%) complain about pain in the paralyzed part(s) of their body, mainly in the upper limbs [35]. Centralized pain is observed in 2–8% of patients. A cross-sectional study by Kong et al. [36] found that, in 42% of stroke patients, ischemic and hemorrhagic pain was sustained in paralyzed limbs.

This led to decreased HRQoL in terms of self-rated physical health at ≥ 6 months as measured using SF-36.

In light of these data, the importance of primary prevention of stroke is obvious. Beyond learning how stroke influences HRQoL, it is also necessary to know how different prophylactic methods influence QoL. This is because some patients may rate their "objective" level of functioning and risk differently.

AF increases the risk of stroke; primary prevention requires taking anticoagulants. In one of the few studies dealing with this topic, only 10% of physicians felt that anticoagulation therapy significantly influenced the HRQoL of patients. Interestingly, they used this therapy more often in younger patients, in whom the risks of anticoagulation therapy outweigh expected benefits (i.e., reducing the chance of a cerebrovascular incident). In another study using patient preferences, based on "the standard gamble" and "the time trade-off" technique, those with AF experienced a mild worsening of HRQoL as a result of using oral anticoagulants [37]. Conversely, the Boston Area Anticoagulation Trial in Atrial Fibrillation (BAATAF) did not observe an influence of anticoagulation therapy on self-rated HRQoL [38]. It did, however, observe a greater incidence of bleeding. By summarizing these few studies, one may conclude that the primary prevention of stroke in AF patients yields a negative influence on HRQoL due to complications related to bleeding. The inconvenience of frequent follow-up visits, regular blood tests, and restrictions in everyday life may also be related to the decreased HRQoL of patients using long-term anticoagulation therapy.

The frequency of stroke rises in accordance with increases in blood pressure. Several randomized clinical studies have found that decreasing blood pressure is associated with a reduced risk for stroke, on average by 30–40%. These observations relate equally to subjects with mild hypertension [39], older individuals [40], isolated systolic hypertension [41], and concomitant DM. A detailed discussion concerning the influence of hypertension treatment on HRQoL – especially important if using pharmacotherapy to treat hypertension as part of primary prevention of stroke – is presented in Chapter 2.

Carotid artery angioplasty and surgical endarterectomy are additional ways of preventing stroke. They work by removing hemodynamically significant stenotic segments of the carotid arteries. Both interventions decrease the long-term risk of stroke in select population groups. One recent study observed significant cognitive dysfunction and decreased HRQoL in 40% of TIA patients and 70% of stroke patients who had their incidents attributed to significant stenosis of the internal carotid artery [42]. In contrast, improvement in cognitive functioning was noted in a group of patients under observation for 1.5 years who did not exhibit new neurological complaints.

The endarterectomy or angioplasty of stenotic carotid arteries may lead to material breaking away from atherosclerotic plaques and entering the cerebral circulation, causing microemboli. Lloyd et al. [43] studied this phenomenon. After following up patients with microemboli resulting from endarterectomy for 6 months and using CT, they did not find it to be a risk factor for cognitive dysfunction, nor did it negatively influence their self-rated HRQoL. Recently, a few systems to prevent the occurrence of cerebral macroemboli and microemboli have started to used in angioplasty.

Nevertheless, there remains a relative lack of large-scale HRQoL studies on patients undergoing carotic artery angioplasty incorporating these temporary protective mechanisms. For instance, Pieniazek et al. [44] conducted a study in 210 patients who, due to carotid artery stenosis, underwent angioplasty with stenting. In this study, 45% of patients had previously suffered a stroke. This study measured the degree of disability (Modified Rankin Scale) and cognitive functioning (MMSE) before and after carotid artery angioplasty, in which proximal and distal cerebral protection was used. Directly after the procedure, worsened cognitive functioning was not observed in any group of patients, and the prevalence of neurological complications was very low.

Secondary prevention, undertaken after a cerebrovascular incident, does not differ essentially from the primary-prevention options discussed above. The use of oral anticoagulants (which are more effective than aspirin) is standard treatment for stroke patients with concomitant AF. Aspirin, ticlopidine, clopidogrel, and dipiridamol, if used long-term, have been found to be of similar effectiveness in secondary prevention after an ischemic stroke or a non-embolic TIA. Studies have found that the angiotensin-converting enzyme inhibitor perindopril, especially combined with indapamide [45], angiotensin-II receptor antagonists (candesartan [46] and eprosartan [47]) is effective in the treatment of hypertension after stroke. However, data are lacking to better describe the HRQoL of patients treated for the secondary prevention of stroke.

8.7 Influence of Stroke on the HRQoL of the Families and Caregivers of Patients

Determining the influence of stroke on the QoL of the families and caregivers of patients is important for various reasons. Firstly, the HRQoL of caregivers is associated with the quality of the care offered to patients in terms of rehabilitation time and material situations. Secondly, stroke requires additional care; it affects the family not only physically, but also psychologically. Chronic stress, tension, organizational difficulties, and little support from the patient/partner add to the exhaustion, lost hope, and often chronic depression in individuals offering care [48].

A few studies have attempted to separate the factors associated with the HRQoL of those looking after stroke patients. Feelings of incompetence, not being able to express negative emotions or adequately deal with stress, restrictions placed on social roles and lifestyle, problems with one's own physical and psychological health, as well as low economic status all add to the decreased HRQoL of caregivers [49]. An additional difficulty of those looking after stroke patients is that they begin to observe in themselves the same problems as the patient, but value them differently [5]. Approximately 80% of the spouses of stroke patients' noted decreased HRQoL in one or more dimensions and 52% suffered from depression.

Different intervention programs aimed at improving knowledge and how to deal with stress in the caregivers of stroke patients may lead to decreased stress and improved HRQoL. The influence of stroke on the HRQoL of caregivers is measured using several questionnaires.

The satisfaction with life felt by the spouses of stroke patients is decreased. Shortly after the incident, their professional status worsens and they are subject to chronic stress. Also negatively affected is their ability to relax, sexual life, and marital relationship. This state is maintained normally for ≤ 1 year after the stroke of their partner [50] and later stabilizes or improves. The spouses of stroke patients whose mobility has been affected, who report sensory problems, and who prevent the patient from living independently rate their HRQoL as low mainly due to exhaustion brought on by obligations, poor sexual life, and problems in the marital relationship. Also, the spouses of patients with cognitive dysfunction and astheno-emotional syndrome are less satisfied with their marital relationship and the quality of their family and sexual life, all of which influence their self-rated HRQoL.

8.8 Conclusions

Stroke and its consequences constitute an important problem for the patient, his/her family, and the healthcare system. Measuring HRQoL in post-stroke patients is an important addition to conventional evaluations of health status. The main factors influencing decreased HRQoL in patients after stroke are: depression; physical and mental disability; chronic pain; cognitive deficits; disturbances in emotion and self-identity; and social isolation. Self-rated HRQoL is dependent upon current neurological state and the ability to care for one's self. It seems that rehabilitation geared towards increasing the independence of post-stroke patients, decreasing isolation, treating depression, and strengthening social support can contribute to improving HRQoL.

References

1. Truelsen T, Piechowski-Jóźwiak B, Bonita R et al (2006) Stroke incidence and prevalence in Europe: a review of available data. Eur J Neurol 13:581-598
2. Heart disease and stroke statistics - 2010 update: a report from the American Heart Association. Circulation 121:e46-e215
3. Haacke C, Althaus A, Spottke A et al (2006) Long-term outcome after stroke: evaluating health-related quality of life using utility measurements. Stroke 37:193-198
4. Grool AM, van der Graaf Y, Witkamp TD et al (2011) Progression of white matter lesion volume and health-related quality of life in patients with symptomatic atherosclerotic disease: The SMART-MR Study. J Aging Res, doi: 10.4061/2011/280630
5. Hochstenbach J, Prigatano G, Mulder T (2005) Patients' and relatives' reports of disturbances 9 months after stroke: subjective changes in physical functioning, cognition, emotion, and behavior. Arch Phys Med Rehab 86:1587-1593
6. Ivan CS, Seshadri S, Beiser A et al (2004) Dementia after stroke: the Framingham Study. Stroke 35:1264-1268
7. Dhamoon MS, Moon YP, Paik MC et al (2009) Long-term functional recovery after first ischemic stroke: The Northern Manhattan Study. Stroke 40:2805–2811
8. Anderson CS, Carter KN, Brownlee WJ et al (2004) Very long-term outcome after stroke in Auckland, New Zealand. Stroke 35:1920-1924
9. Hackett ML, Duncan JR, Anderson CS et al (2000) Health-related quality of life among long-term survivors of stroke: results from the Auckland Stroke Study, 1991-1992. Stroke 31:440-447
10. Torrance GW (1987) Utility approach to measuring health-related quality of life. J Chron Dis 40:593-600
11. Post PN, Stiggelbout AM, Wakker PP (2001) The utility of health states after stroke. Stroke 32:1425 1429
12. Sturm JW, Osborne RH, Dewey HM et al (2002) Brief comprehensive quality of life assessment after stroke: the assessment of quality of life instrument in the north East Melbourne stroke incidence study (NEMESIS). Stroke 33:2888-2894
13. Ahmed S, Mayo NE, Corbiere M (2005) Change in quality of life of people with stroke over time: True change or response shift? Qual Life Res 14:611-627
14. Pickard AS, Johnson JA, Feeny DH (2005) Responsiveness of generic health-related quality of life measures in stroke. Qual Life Res 14:207-219
15. Toso V, Gandolfo C, Paolucci S et al (2004) Post-stroke depression: research methodology of a large multicentre observational study (DESTRO). Neurol Sci 25:138-144
16. Hackett ML, Yapa C, Parag V et al (2005) Frequency of depression after stroke: a systematic review of observational studies. Stroke 36:1330-1340
17. Kim JS, Choi KS (2000) Poststroke depression and emotional incontinence: correlation with lesion location. Neurology 54:1805-1810
18. Moon Y-S, Kim S-J, Kim H-C et al (2004) Correlates of quality of life after stroke. J Neurol Sci 224:37-41

19. Hilari K, Byng S, Lamping DL et al (2003) Stroke and Aphasia Quality of Life Scale-39 (SAQOL-39): evaluation of acceptability, reliability, and validity. Stroke 34:1944-1950
20. Carlsson GE, Moller A, Blomstrand C (2004) A qualitative study of the consequences of 'hidden dysfunctions' one year after a mild stroke in persons < 75 years. Disabil Rehabil 26:1373-1380
21. Sturm JW, Donnan GA, Dewey HM et al (2004) Quality of life after stroke: the North East Melbourne Stroke Incidence Study (NEMESIS). Stroke 35:2340-2345
22. Kapral MK, Fang J, Hill MD et al (2005) Investigators of the Registry of the Canadian Stroke Network: Sex differences in stroke care and outcomes: results from the Registry of the Canadian Stroke Network. Stroke 36:809-814
23. Nichols-Larsen DS, Clark PC, Zeringue A et al (2005) Factors influencing stroke survivors' quality of life during subacute recovery. Stroke 36:1480-1484
24. Van Exel NJ, Scholte op Reimer WJ, Koopmanschap MA (2004) Assessment of post-stroke quality of life in cost-effectiveness studies: the usefulness of the Barthel Index and the EuroQoL-5D. Qual Life Res 13:427-433
25. Jonsson AC, Lindgren I, Hallstrom B et al (2005) Determinants of quality of life in stroke survivors and their informal caregivers. Stroke 36:803-808
26. Bluvol A, Ford-Gilboe M (2004) Hope, health work and quality of life in families of stroke survivors. J Advanc Nurs 48:322-332
27. Paul SL, Sturm JW, Dewey HM et al (2005) Long-term outcome in the North East Melbourne Stroke Incidence Study: predictors of quality of life at 5 years after stroke. Stroke 36:2082-2086
28. Kase CS, Wolf PA, Kelly-Hayes M et al (1998) Intellectual decline after stroke: the Framingham Study. Stroke 29:805-812
29. Araki A, Murotani Y, Kamimiya F, Ito H (2004) Low well-being is an independent predictor for stroke in elderly patients with diabetes mellitus. J Am Geriatr Soc 52:205-210
30. Agewall S, Wilkstrand J, Fagerberg B (1998) Stroke was predicted by dimensions of quality of life in treated hypertensive men. Stroke 29:2329-2333
31. Schindler RJ (2005) Dementia with cerebrovascular disease: the benefits of early treatment. Eur J Neurol 12, suppl. 3:17-21
32. Choi-Kwon S, Han SW, Kwon SU et al (2005) Poststroke fatigue: characteristics and related factors. Cerebrovasc Dis 19:84-90
33. Glader EL, Stegmayr B, Asplund K (2002) Poststroke fatigue: a 2-year follow-up of stroke patients in Sweden. Stroke 33:1327-1333
34. Bogusslavsky J, Straub F (2003) Disabling fatigue after full recovery from stroke. Stroke 34:317-318
35. Bender L, McKenna K (2001) Hemiplegic shoulder pain: defining the problem and its management. Disabil Rehabil 16:698-705
36. Kong K-H, Woon V-C, Yang S-Y (2004) Prevalence of chronic pain and its impact on health-related quality of life in stroke survivors. Arch Phys Med Rehabil 85:35-40
37. Gage BF, Cardinalli AB, Owens DK (1996) The effect of stroke and stroke prophylaxis with aspirin or warfarin on quality of life. Arch Intern Med 156:1829-1836
38. Lancaster TR, Singer DE, Sheehan MA et al (1991) The impact of long-term warfarin therapy on quality of life – the Boston Area Anticoagulation Trial for Atrial Fibrillation Investigation. Arch Intern Med 15:1944-1949
39. Hansson L, Zanchetti A, Carruthers SG et al (1998) Effects of intensive blood-pressure lowering and low-dose aspirin in patients with hypertension: principal results of the Hypertension Optimal Treatment (HOT) randomized trial. Lancet 351:1755-1762
40. Beckett NS, Peters R, Fletcher AE et al (2008) Treatment of hypertension in patients 80 years of age or older. N Engl J Med 358:1887-1898
41. Staessen JA, Fagard R, Thijs L et al (1997) Randomised double-blind comparison of placebo and active treatment for older patients with isolated systolic hypertension. Lancet 350:757-764

42. Bakker FC, Klijn CJ, van der Grond J (2004) Cognition and quality of life in patients with carotid artery occlusion: a follow-up study. Neurology 62:2230-2235
43. Lloyd AJ, Hayes PD, London NJ (2004) Does carotid endarterectomy lead to a decline in cognitive function or health related quality of life? J Clin Exper Neuropsychol 26:817-825
44. Pieniążek P, Musiałek P, Kabłak-Ziembicka A et al (2005) Implantation of stents with the application of proximal and distal protection system of the brain as a new method of treatment of carotid artery stenoses. Post Kardiol Interw 1:16-24
45. PROGRESS Collaborative group (2001) Randomised trial of perindopril-based blood pressure-lowering regimen among 6105 individuals with previous stroke or transient ischaemic attack. Lancet 358:1033-1041
46. Schrader J, Luders S, Kulschewski A et al (2003) The ACCESS Study: evaluation of acute candesartan cilexetil therapy in stroke survivors. Stroke 34:1699-1703
47. Schrader J, Luders S, Kulschewski A et al (2005) Morbidity and mortality after stroke, eprosartan compared with nitrendipine for secondary prevention: principal results of a prospective randomized controlled study (MOSES). Stroke 36:1218-1226
48. Lynch EB, Butt Z, Heinemann A et al (2008) A qualitative study of quality of life after stroke: the importance of social relationships. J Rehabil Med 40:518-523
49. Visser-Meily A, Post M, Riphagen II et al (2004) Measures used to assess burden among caregivers of stroke patients: a review. Clin Rehabil 18:601 623
50. Forsberg-Warleby G, Moller A, Blomstrand C (2004) Life satisfaction in spouses of patients with stroke during the first year after stroke. J Rehabil Med 36: 4-11

Appendix: Questionnaires Used for the Assessment of Quality of Life in Patients with Cardiovascular Diseases with Relevant References

Marek Klocek

1. The Most Often Used Generic Quality of Life Questionnaires

Nottingham Health Profile (NHP)

Hunt SM, McKenna SP, McEwen J et al (1980) A quantitative approach to perceived health status: a validation study. J Epidemiol Comm Health 34:281–286

Herlitz J, Brandrup-Wognsen G, Evander MH et al (2009) Quality of life 15 years after coronary artery bypass grafting. Coron Artery Dis 20:363–369

Short Form Health Survey 36 (SF-36)

Anderson CS, Laubscher S, Burns R (1996) Validation of the short form 36 (SF-36) health survey questionnaire among stroke patients. Stroke 27:1812–1816

Ware JE Jr, Kosinski M, Bayliss MS et al (1995) Comparison of methods for the scoring and statistical analysis of SF-36 health profile and summary measures: summary of results from the Medical Outcomes Study. Med Care 33:AS264–A279

Filade I, Ramos I (2000) Validity and reliability of the SF-36 Health Survey Questionnaire in patients with coronary artery disease. J Clin Epidemiol 53:359–365

Short Form Health Survey 12 (SF-12)

Ware J, Kosiniski M, Keller SD (1996) A 12-item Short-Form Health Survey (SF-12): construction of scales and preliminary tests of reliability and validity. Med Care 34:220–233

Muller-Nordhorn J, Nolte CH, Rossnagel K et al (2005) The use of the 12-item short-form health status instrument in a longitudinal study of patients with stroke and transient ischaemic attack. Neuroepidemiology 24:196-202

M. Klocek (✉)
I Department of Cardiology and Hypertension
Jagiellonian University Medical College, Kraków, Poland
e-mail: marek.klocek@wp.pl

K. Kawecka-Jaszcz et al. (eds.), *Health-Related Quality of Life in Cardiovascular Patients*,
DOI: 10.1007/978-88-470-2769-5_9 © Springer-Verlag Italia 2013

Sickness Impact Profile (SIP)

Schuling J, Greidanus J, Meyboom-De Jong B (1993) Measuring functional status of stroke patients with the Sickness Impact Profile. Disabil Rehabil 15:19–23

2. The Most Often Used Disease- or Problem-Specific Quality of Life Questionnaires

Angina Pectoris Quality of Life Questionnaire (AQLQ)

Wiklund I, Comerford MB, Dimenäs E (1991) The relationship between exercise tolerance and quality of life in angina pectoris. Clin Cardiol 14:204–208

Angina-Related Limitations at Work Questionnaire

Lerner DJ, Amick III BC, Malspeis S et al (1998) The Angina-related Limitations at Work Questionnaire. Qual Life Res 7:23–32

Atrial Fibrillation Severity Scale

Bubien RS, Knotts-Dolson SM, Plumb VJ et al (1996) Effect of radiofrequency catheter ablation on health-related quality of life and activities of daily living in patients with recurrent arrhythmias. Circulation 94:1585–1591

Barthel Index (BI)

Mahoney F, Barthel D (1965) Functional evaluation: the Barthel index. Md State Med J 14:61–65

van Exel NJA, Scholte op Reimer WJM, Koopmanschap MA (2004) Assessment of post-stroke quality of life in cost-effectiveness studies: The usefulness of the Barthel Index and the EuroQoL-5D. Qual Life Res 13:427–433

Beck Depression Scale

Beck A, Mendelson M, Mock J (1961) Inventory for measuring depression. Arch Gen Psychiatry 4:561–571

Burden of Stroke Scale (BOSS)

Doyle PJ, McNeil MR, Mikolic JM et al (2004) The Burden of Stroke Scale (BOSS) provides valid and reliable score estimates of functioning and well-being in stroke survivors with and without communication disorders. J Clin Epidemiol 57:997–1007

Cardiac Health Profile (CHP)

Kiessling A, Henriksson P (2004) Perceived cognitive function is a major determinant of health related quality of life in a non-selected population of patients with coronary artery disease – a principal components analysis. Qual Life Res 13:1621–1631

Wahrborg P, Emanuelsson H (1996) The Cardiac Health Profile: content, reliability and validity of a new disease-specific quality of life questionnaire. Coron Artery Dis 7:823–829

Cardiovascular Limitations and Symptoms Profile (CLASP)

Lewin RJ, Thompson DR, Martin CR et al (2002) Validation of the Cardiovascular Limitations and Symptoms Profile (CLASP) in chronic stable angina. J Cardiopulm Rehabil 22:184–191

Chronic Heart Failure Questionnaire (CHQ)

Guyatt GH, Nogradi S, Halcrow S (1989) Development and testing of a new measure of health status for clinical trials in heart failure. J Gen Intern Med 4:101–107

Wyrwich KW, Spertus JA, Kroenke K (2004) Heart Disease Expert Panel. Clinically important differences in health status for patients with heart disease: an expert consensus panel report. Am Heart J 147:615–622

Duke Health Profile (DHP)

Parkerson GR, Broadhead WE, Tse C-KJ (1990) The Duke Health Profile: a 17-item measure of health and dysfunction. Med Care 28:1056–1069

Perret-Guillaume C, Briancon S, Guillemin F et al (2010) Which generic health related Quality of Life questionnaire should be used in older inpatients: comparison of the Duke Health Profile and the MOS Short-Form SF-36? J Nutr Health Aging 14:325–331

European Heart Failure Self-Care Behavior Scale (EHFScBS)

Jaarsma T, Stromberg A, Martensson J et al (2003) Development and testing of the European Heart Failure Self-Care Behaviour Scale. Eur J Heart Failure 5:363–370

Cameron J, Worrall-Carter L, Driscoll A et al (2009) Measuring self-care in chronic heart failure: a review of the psychometric properties of clinical instruments. J Cardiovasc Nurs 24:E10–E22

Jaarsma T, Arestedt KF, Mårtensson J et al (2009) The European Heart Failure Self-care Behaviour scale revised into a nine-item scale (EHFScB-9): a reliable and valid international instrument. Eur J Heart Fail 11:99–105

EuroQoL-5D (EQ-5D)

Dorman PJ, Waddel F, Slattery J et al (1997) Are proxy assessment of health status after stroke with the Euro-HRQoL Questionnaire feasible, accurate and unbiased? Stroke 28:1883–1887

Dorman PJ, Waddel F, Slattery J et al (1997) Is the Euro-HRQoL a valid measure of health-related quality of life after stroke. Stroke 28:1876–1882

Dorman PJ, Dennis M, Sandercock P (1999) How do scores on the EuroQol relate to scores on the SF-36 after stroke? Stroke 30:2146–2151

van Exel NJ, Scholte op Reimer WJ, Koopmanschap MA (2004) Assessment of post-stroke quality of life in cost-effectiveness studies: the usefulness of the Barthel Index and the EuroQoL-5D. Qual Life Res 13:427–433

Nowels D, McGloin J, Westfall JM et al (2005) Validation of the EQ-5D quality of life instrument in patients after myocardial infarction. Qual Life Res 14:95–105

Health Complaints Scale in Coronary Artery Disease (HCS-CAD)

Pedersen SS, Denollet J (2002) Perceived health following myocardial infarction: cross-validation of the Health Complaints Scale in Danish patients. Behav Res Ther 40:1221–1230

Pelle AJ, Pedersen SS, Erdman RA et al (2011) Anhedonia is associated with poor health status and more somatic and cognitive symptoms in patients with coronary artery disease. Qual Life Res 20:643–651

Health Utilities Index (HUI)

Mathias SD, Bates MM, Pasta DJ et al (1997) Use of Health Utilities Index with stroke patients and their caregivers. Stroke 28:1888–1894

Furlong WJ, Feeny DH, Torrance GW et al (2001) The Health Utilities Index (HUI) system for assessing health-related quality of life in clinical studies. Ann Med 33:375–384

Pickard AS, Johnson JA, Feeny DH et al (2004) Agreement between patient and proxy assessment of health-related quality of life after stroke using EQ-5D and Health Utilities Index. Stroke 35:607–612

International Index of Erectile Dysfunction (IIEF-5)

Rosen RC, Cappelleri JC, Smith MD (1999) Development and evaluation of a abridged, 5-item version of the International Index of Erectile Function (IIEF-5) as a diagnostic tool for erectile dysfunction. Int J Impot Res 11:319–326

Kansas City Cardiomyopathy Questionnaire

Green CP, Porter CB, Bresnahan DR et al (2000) Development and evaluation of the Kansas City Cardiomyopathy Questionnaire: a new health status measure for heart failure. J Am Coll Cardiol 35:1245–1255

Pettersen KI, Reikvam A, Rollag A et al (2005) Reliability and validity of the Kansas City Cardiomyopathy Questionnaire in patients with previous myocardial infarction. Eur J Heart Fail 7:235–242

Karnofsky Performance Scale (KPS)

Karnofsky DA (1961) Meaningful clinical classification of therapeutic responses to anticancer drugs. Clin Pharmacol Ther 2:709–717

Mor V, Laliberte L, Morris JN et al (1984) The Karnofsky Performance Status Scale. An examination of its reliability and validity in a research setting. Cancer 53:2002–2007

Karolinska Questionnaire

Levy T, Walker S, Rex S et al (2000) Ablate and pace for drug refractory paroxysmal atrial fibrillation. Is ablation necessary? Int J Cardiol 75:187–195

Left Ventricular Dysfunction Questionnaire (LVD-36)

O'Leary C, Jones P (2000) The left ventricular dysfunction questionnaire (LVD-36): reliability, validity and responsiveness. Heart 83:634–640

London Handicap Scale

Harwood RW, Gompertz P, Ebrahim S (1994) Handicap one year after a stroke: validity of a new scale. J Neurol Neurosurg Psych 57:825–828

MacNew Heart Disease Health-Related Quality of Life Questionnaire (MacNew)

Dixon T, Lim LL, Oldridge NB (2002) The MacNew heart disease health-related quality of life instrument: Reference data for users. Qual Life Res 11:173–183

McMasters Health Index Questionnaire

Chambers LN, MacDonald LA, Tugwell P et al (1982) The McMaster Health Index questionnaire as a measure of the quality of life for patients with rheumatic disease. J Reumatol 90:780–784

de Haan R, Aaronson N, Limburg M et al (1993) Measuring quality of life in stroke. Stroke 24:320–327

Minnesota Living with Heart Failure Questionnaire (MLHF-Q)

Middel B, Bouma J, de Jongste M et al (2001) Psychometric properties of the Minnesota Living with Heart Failure Questionnaire (MLHF-Q). Clin Rehabil 15:489–500

Riegel B, Moser D, Glaser D et al (2002) The Minnesota Living with Heart Failure Questionnaire: sensitivity to differences and responsiveness to intervention intensity in a clinical population. Nurs Res 51:209–218

Hak T, Willems D, van der Wal G et al (2004) A qualitative validation of the Minnesota Living with Heart Failure Questionnaire. Qual Life Res 13:417–426

Mini Mental State Examination (MMSE)

Tombaugh TN, McIntyre NJ (1992) The mini-mental state examination: a comprehensive review. J Am Geriatr Soc 40:922–935

Molloy DW, Standish TI (1997) A guide to the standardized Mini-Mental State Examination. Int Psychogeriatr 9 (Suppl 1):87–94

Minor Symptom Evaluation Profile (MSEP)

Walle PO, Westergren G, Dimenas E et al (1994) Effects of 100 mg of controlled-release metoprolol and 100 mg of atenolol on blood pressure, central nervous system-related symptoms, and general well being. J Clin Pharmacol 34:742–747

Modified Rankin Scale (mRS)

Sulter G, Steen C, De KJ (1999) Use of the Barthel index and modified Rankin scale in acute stroke trials. Stroke 30:1538–1541

Banks JL, Marotta CA (2007) Outcomes validity and reliability of the modified Rankin scale: implications for stroke clinical trials: a literature review and synthesis. Stroke 38:1091–1096

Myocardial Infarction Dimensional Assessment Scale (MIDAS)

Thompson DR, Jenkinson C, Roebuck A et al (2002) Development and validation of a short measure of health status for individuals with acute myocardial infarction: the Myocardial Infarction Dimensional Assessment Scale (MIDAS). Qual Life Res 11:535–543

Newcastle Stroke-Specific Quality of Life Measure (NEWSQOL)

Buck D, Jacoby A, Massey A et al (2004) Development and validation of NEWSQOL, the Newcastle Stroke-Specific Quality of Life Measure. Cerebrovasc Dis 17:143–152

Baumann M, Lurbe K, Leandro ME et al (2012) Life satisfaction of two-year post-stroke survivors: effects of socio-economic factors, motor impairment, Newcastle stroke-specific quality of life measure and world health organization quality of life: bref of informal caregivers in Luxembourg and a rural area in Portugal. Cerebrovasc Dis 33:219–230

Pacemaker Symptom Scale

Menozzi C, Brignole M, Moracchini PV, Lolli G, Bacchi M, Tesorieri MC, Tosoni GD, Bollini R (1990) Intrapatient comparison between chronic VVIR and DDD pacing in patients affected by high degree AV block without heart failure. Pacing Clin Electrophysiol 13:1816–1822

Psychological General Well Being Index (PGWB)

Dupuy HJ (1984) The Psychological General Well-Being (PGWB) Index. In: Wenger NK, Mattson ME, Furberg CF, Elison J (ed) Assessment of quality of life in clinical trials of cardiovascular therapies. Le Jacq Publishing, Shelton, CT, pp 170–183

Wilkund IK, Halling K, Ryden-Bergsten T et al (1997) Does lowering the blood pressure improve the mood? Quality-of-life results from the Hypertension Optimal Treatment (HOT) Study. Blood Pres 6:357–364

Quality of Life After Myocardial Infarction (QLMI)

Hillers TK, Guyatt GH, Oldridge N et al (1994) Quality of life after myocardial infarction. J Clin Epidemiol 47:1287–1296

Quality of Life Index

Ferrans CE, Powers MJ (1985) Quality of Life Index: development and psychometric properties. ANS Ad Nurs Sci 8:15–24

Quality of Life Index - Cardiac Version III

Dougherty CM, Dewhurst T, Nichol WP et al (1998) Comparison of three quality of life instruments in stable angina pectoris: Seattle Angina Questionnaire, Short Form Health Survey (SF-36), and Quality of Life Index-Cardiac Version III. J Clin Epidemiol 51:569–575

Quality of Life in Severe Heart Failure Questionnaire (QLQ-SHF)

Berry C, McMurray J (1999) A review of quality of life evaluations in patients with congestive heart failure. PharmacoEconomics 16:247–271

Wiklund I, Waagstein F, Swedberg K et al (1996) Quality of life on treatment with metropolol in dilated cardiomyopathy: results from the MDC trial. Cardiovasc Drugs Ther 10:361–368

Quality of Well-being Scale (QWB)

Ganiats TG, Palinkas LA, Kaplan RM (1992) Comparison of Quality of Well-Being scale and Functional Status Index in patients with atrial fibrillation. Med Care 30:958–964

Ganiats TG, Browner DK, Dittrich HC (1998) Comparison of Quality of Well-Being scale and NYHA functional status classification in patients with atrial fibrillation. Am Heart J 135:819–824

Reitan Trail-making Test (RTMT)

Reitan RM (1958) Validity of the trail making test as an indicator of organic brain damage. Percept Mot Skills 8:271–276

Schedule for the Evaluation of Individual Quality of Life-Direct Weight (SEIQoL-DW)

LeVasseur SA, Green S, Talman P (2005) The SEIQoL-DW is a valid method for measuring individual quality of life in stroke survivors attending a secondary prevention clinic. Qual Life Res 14:779–788

Seattle Angina Questionnaire (SAQ)

Spertus J (1997) The Seattle Angina Questionnaire: A review of the instrument and its applications. Qual Life Newsletter 16:9–11

Dougherty CM, Dewhurst T, Nichol WP et al (1998) Comparison of three quality of life instruments in stable angina pectoris: the Seattle Angina Questionnarie (SAQ), the Short Form Health Survey (SF-36) and the Quality of Life Index-Cardiac Version III (QLI). J Clin Epidemiol 51:569–575

Specific Activity Scale (SAS)

Brignole M, Gianfranchi L, Menozzi C et al (1994) Influence of atrioventricular junction radiofrequency ablation in patients with chronic atrial fibrillation and flutter on quality of life and cardiac performance. Am J Cardiol 74:242–246

Stroke Adapted Sickness Impact Profile (SA-SIP30)

van Straten A, de Haan RJ, Limburg M et al (1997) A stroke-adapted 30-item version of the Sickness Impact Profile to assess quality of life (SA-SIP30). Stroke 28:2155–2161

van Straten A, de Haan RJ, Limburg M et al (2000) Clinical meaning of the Stroke-Adapted Sickness Impact profile-30 and the Sickness Impact Profile-136. Stroke 31:2610–2615

Stroke Impact Scale (SIS)

Studenski S, Duncan PW, Perera S et al (2005) Daily functioning and quality of life in a randomized controlled trial of therapeutic exercise for subacute stroke survivors. Stroke 36:1764–1770

Duncan PW, Wallace D, Lai SM et al (1999) The Stroke Impact Scale version 2.0: evaluation of reliability, validity, and sensitivity to change. Stroke 30:2131–2140

Stroke Specific Quality of Life Scale (SS-QoL Scale)

Williams LS, Weinberger M, Harris LE et al (1999) Development of a Stroke-Specific Quality of Life Scale. Stroke 30:1362–1369

Muus I, Ringsberg KC (2005) Stroke Specific Quality of Life Scale: Danish adaptation and a pilot study for testing psychometric properties. Scand J Caring Sci 19:140–147

Subjective Symptoms Assessment Profile (SSA-P)

Dimenas ES, Dalhof C, Olofsson B et al (1990) An instrument for quantifying subjective symptoms among untreated and treated hypertensives: development and documentation. J Clin Res Pharmacoepid 4:205–217

Kawecka-Jaszcz K, Czarnecka D, Klocek M et al (2006) Rilmenidine – its antihypertensive efficacy, safety and impact on quality of life in perimenopausal women with mild to moderate essential hypertension. Blood Press 15:51–58

Symptom Checklist (SCL)

Kang Y, Bahler R (2004) Health-related quality of life in patients newly diagnosed with atrial fibrillation. Eur J Cardiovasc Nurs 3:71–76

Reynolds MR, Lavelle T, Essebag V (2006) Influence of age, sex, and atrial fibrillation recurrence on quality of life outcomes in a population of patients with new-onset atrial fibrillation: the Fibrillation Registry Assessing Costs, Therapies, Adverse events and Lifestyle (FRACTAL) study. Am Heart J 152:1097–1103

Symptom Questionnaire for Hypertensive Patients

Bulpitt C, Dollery C, Carne S (1974) A symptom questionnaire for hypertensive patients. J Chron Dis 27:309–323

Bulpitt C, Fletcher A (1990) The measurement of quality of life in hypertensive patients: a practical approach. Br J Clin Pharmacol 30:353–364

Vital Signs Quality of Life Questionnaire (VSQLQ)

Kong BW, Bean JA, Stephens D (1995) Assessment of the Vital Signs Quality of Life Questionnaire in three studies on hypertension. J Hum Hypertens 9:255–262

Leidy NK, Schmier JK, Bonomi AE et al (2000) Psychometric properties of the VSQLQ in black patients with mild hypertension. Vital Signs Quality of Life Questionnaire. J Nation Med Ass 92:550–557

Zung Depression Scale

Zung WWK (1965) A self-rating depression scale. Arch Gen Psych 12:67–70

Biggs JT, Wylie LT, Ziegler VE (1978) Validity of the Zung Self-rating Depression Scale. Br J Psychiatry 132:381–385

Index

K. Kawecka-Jaszcz et al. (eds.), *Health-Related Quality of Life in Cardiovascular Patients*,
DOI: 10.1007/978-88-470-2769-5 © Springer-Verlag Italia 2013

N

O

P

Q

R

S

Printed in August 2012

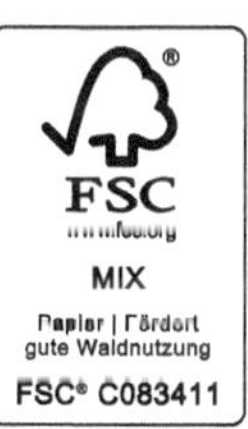

Zeitfracht Medien GmbH
Ferdinand-Jühlke-Straße 7
99095 Erfurt, Deutschland
produktsicherheit@kolibri360.de